# THE PTSD SOLUTION

*Your Complete Guide to Overcome the Behaviors that Keep You Trapped, Break the Cycle of Fear, Manage Trauma, and Find Peace*

J.G. HOXIE

© **Copyright J.G. Hoxie - 2025 - All rights reserved.**

The content within this book may not be reproduced, duplicated or transmitted without direct written permission from the author or the publisher.

Under no circumstances will any blame or legal responsibility be held against the publisher, or author, for any damages, reparation, or monetary loss due to the information contained within this book. Either directly or indirectly. You are responsible for your own choices, actions, and results.

**Legal Notice:**

This book is copyright protected. This book is only for personal use. You cannot amend, distribute, sell, use, quote or paraphrase any part, of the content within this book, without the consent of the author or publisher.

**Disclaimer Notice:**

Please note the information contained within this document is for educational and entertainment purposes only. All effort has been expended to present accurate, up-to-date, and reliable, complete information. No warranties of any kind are declared or implied. Readers acknowledge that the author is not engaging in the rendering of legal, financial, medical or professional advice. The content within this book has been derived from various sources. Please consult a licensed professional before attempting any techniques outlined in this book.

By reading this document, the reader agrees that under no circumstances is the author responsible for any losses, direct or indirect, which are incurred as a result of the use of the information contained within this document, including, but not limited to, — errors, omissions, or inaccuracies.

# TABLE OF CONTENTS

| | |
|---|---|
| Introduction | 7 |
| **1. UNDERSTANDING YOUR PTSD** | 11 |
| Demystifying PTSD: Beyond the Diagnoses | 11 |
| The Science Behind Trauma: What Happens in Your Brain | 13 |
| Recognizing Symptoms: The Silent Impacts on Daily Life | 15 |
| Intersectional Insights: How Culture and Gender Shape PTSD | 18 |
| The Therapeutic Alliance: Finding the Right Support | 20 |
| Dealing with the Mental Health System: Your Essential Guide | 22 |
| **2. BUILDING A FOUNDATION OF SELF-COMPASSION** | 25 |
| What is Self-Compassion? | 25 |
| Overcoming Self-Criticism: Your Inner Dialogue | 28 |
| Practical Exercises for Daily Self-Compassion | 30 |
| Mindfulness and Self-Acceptance: A Dual Approach | 32 |
| Journaling for Healing: Writing Your Path to Recovery | 34 |
| Creating a Safe Space: Your Sanctuary for Growth | 37 |
| **3. DEALING WITH EMOTIONAL TURBULENCE** | 41 |
| How to Cope With Triggers | 41 |
| Grounding Techniques: Staying Present in the Now | 45 |
| Managing Flashbacks: Techniques for Immediate Relief | 47 |
| Emotional Regulation: Balancing Your Inner World | 49 |
| The Power of Breath: Breathing Exercises for Calm | 52 |
| Anger Management: Reframing Intense Emotions | 54 |
| **4. PRACTICAL COPING STRATEGIES FOR EVERYDAY LIFE** | 57 |
| The Importance of a Daily Routine | 57 |
| Mindful Mornings: Setting the Tone for Your Day | 60 |

| | |
|---|---|
| Workplace Strategies: Dealing with Triggers in Professional Settings | 62 |
| Social Situations: Preparing for Potential Challenges | 64 |
| Sleep Solutions: Overcoming Nightmares and Insomnia | 66 |
| Nutrition and Physical Health: Supporting Your Mind Through Body | 69 |

5. REBUILDING RELATIONSHIPS AND COMMUNITY 73
   How to Establish Open and Clear Communication 73
   Trust and Intimacy: Re-Establishing Connections 76
   Gender-Specific Challenges in Relationships 78
   Building Your Support Network: Finding Your Tribe 80
   The Role of Online Communities in Healing 82
   Healing with Empathy: Helping Others Understand What You're Going Through 83

6. HARNESSING THE POWER OF NARRATIVE AND STORYTELLING 85
   Sharing Your Story 86
   Storytelling Workshops: Creating Your Narrative 88
   Creating a Narrative Worth Telling 89
   Writing as Therapy: Unleashing Your Inner Author 90
   Changing Trauma into Triumph 92

7. LONG-TERM WELLNESS AND RESILIENCE 95
   Resilience in Everyday Life 95
   Preparing for Potential Relapses: Strategies for Stability 98
   Creating a Balance: Integrating Work, Life, and Healing 100
   Empowerment Through Self-Advocacy: Claiming Your Rights 103
   Celebrating Progress: Acknowledging Your Achievements 105

8. LOOK TOWARD A HOLISTIC APPROACH TO HEALING 109
   How Your Emotions Impact Your Health 110
   Integrating Yoga and Movement: A Path to Serenity 112
   Meditation Practices: Finding Peace Within 114
   Mindful Eating: Feeding Your Brain 116

| | |
|---|---|
| Engaging in Creative Therapies: Art and Music | 117 |
| Creative Artistic Therapy Options | 119 |
| Conclusion | 121 |
| References | 125 |

# INTRODUCTION

Fight or flight ... do you know the feeling? Your heart starts to race, your chest feels heavy, and a light, almost imperceptible sweat starts —perhaps at the base of your neck, your brow, your top lip? Then, the shaking begins. But why?

Because something deep inside your psyche has been triggered— maybe it was a siren blaring, a loud noise out of place on Sunday morning, the smell of fire, or simply some bad news. Whatever it was, it's taken you back to a moment in time that changed your life, and not for the better. For me, I can name several points in my life that created triggers: my father walking out on our family, an abusive boss (or two, or three), or waking up to my house burning down around me, just to name a few that led me to this important work. So then, the question becomes: How do we battle the triggers of PTSD?

The weight of each day can feel insurmountable for those living with PTSD. This book is for those of us who have experienced trauma and, perhaps like you, seek a path through the darkness.

There's a lot of literature on PTSD, but not enough of it combines empathy with research. Clinical words in a journal can only help so much; you have to understand where people are coming from in order to be able to help.

This work revolves around personal empowerment and emotional healing. I advocate for shadow work—embracing our imperfections rather than trying to fix what isn't broken. We are whole, even when we feel fragmented. This philosophy shapes my approach, where I reject traditional self-help notions and instead focus on self-acceptance and integration.

My goal is to be able to reach all trauma survivors—yourself included. I'm here to address the unique challenges you face and provide tailored content to meet your needs. Together, we can build a sense of understanding and community, reminding you that you are not alone.

A cornerstone of your work here will be self-compassion because you need to treat yourself with kindness and patience. Healing is not a race, and there is no finish line; it's a process, one that requires gentle nurturing and acceptance of where you are without rejecting that in favor of where you want to be. It's important to set realistic expectations because healing from PTSD is always going to be challenging. However, it's also deeply rewarding and filled with catharsis.

I invite you to begin with an open mind and heart. Explore the insights and tools within these pages, and allow yourself to grow and heal. The path ahead may be daunting, but it's also filled with the promise of renewal. Let's work through your healing process together, ready to reclaim resilience and find peace.

*Note:The information provided in this book is intended for educational purposes only and should not be used as a substitute for professional medical advice, diagnosis, or treatment. Working with PTSD and trauma involves deep emotional processing and healing, which may not be suitable for everyone without professional guidance. If you are experiencing mental health challenges or emotional distress, it is important to consult with a qualified healthcare provider, therapist, or mental health professional. The author and publisher of this book disclaim any liability or risk for any direct or indirect consequences resulting from the use or application of any information contained in this book. Always seek the advice of your physician or other qualified health provider with any questions regarding your mental or physical health.*

CHAPTER 1

# UNDERSTANDING YOUR PTSD

When my brother returned home from his deployment, everything seemed different. The once comforting hum of city life had turned into a cacophony of anxiety. Car backfires made his heart race; crowded sidewalks felt suffocating. Jake's experience encapsulates the daily reality for many living with PTSD, a condition that turns the mundane into a battlefield, the mind constantly scanning for threats, either real or imagined. In order to deal with PTSD, we first have to demystify it, shedding light on its complexities and helping you understand that you're not alone in this fight. Together, we'll explore the nuances of PTSD, move beyond the labels, and seek clarity amidst the chaos.

## DEMYSTIFYING PTSD: BEYOND THE DIAGNOSES

PTSD, or post-traumatic stress disorder, moves beyond the confines of clinical definitions and enters the realm of everyday life, an experience that can manifest in countless ways. For some, it might be a sudden flood of memories triggered by a seemingly innocuous sound, like the crack of fireworks echoing the gunfire of a battlefield. For others, it might be the overwhelming sense of dread in a crowded room, where every voice and movement feels like a threat. PTSD infiltrates daily life, altering perceptions and reactions in ways that are as unique as fingerprints (National Institute of Mental Health 2024).

My friend Maria became the survivor of a natural disaster when the Woolsey fire broke out in California in 2018. She now finds herself unable to settle at the sound of wind or even a fire engine, the sense of impending doom setting in and triggering her PTSD. My friend Tom, meanwhile, was in a car accident and now feels his pulse quicken every time he gets behind the wheel. PTSD is not just one thing; those who suffer from it come from diverse backgrounds and experiences, dispelling the myth that this condition only affects combat veterans. PTSD is not limited by profession or circumstance; it touches anyone who has witnessed or endured trauma. This is something you'll need to understand if we're going to break down the misconceptions that often surround this condition.

One of the most damaging misconceptions is the belief that PTSD sufferers are inherently dangerous or unstable. Media portrayals have often sensationalized these narratives—a surefire route to stigma and misunderstanding. However, it's important to recognize that PTSD is a spectrum disorder characterized by a range of symptoms and intensities. For some, it may be relentless nightmares or intrusive thoughts; for others, it might be an undercurrent of anxiety that never quite dissipates. The variability in symptom severity means that each person's experience is different, and this diversity must be acknowledged and respected.

Understanding PTSD also involves distinguishing it from other mental health conditions like anxiety and depression. While there are overlaps, PTSD has unique characteristics, such as re-experiencing symptoms—flashbacks or nightmares that transport you back to the traumatic event. Complex PTSD (CPTSD) adds another layer, often resulting from prolonged exposure to trauma, such as in cases of abuse or captivity. It involves additional symptoms such as emotional dysregulation and a distorted sense of self, which require careful treatment and empathy (Maercker et al. 2022).

Empathy is an extremely important tool in general when it comes to reducing the stigma around PTSD. Creating a culture of understanding allows us to begin to dismantle the barriers that prevent individuals from seeking help. Using empathetic language—such as acknowledging the courage it takes to cope with PTSD daily—can make a significant difference. Instead of viewing those with PTSD as broken, we should celebrate their resilience and strength. Recognizing the role of media in shaping perceptions, it's necessary to challenge inaccuracies and advocate for more nuanced, accurate portrayals.

As we work through the intricacies of PTSD together, remember that empathy and knowledge are powerful allies. Whether you're seeking to understand your own experiences or those of a loved one, this exploration is a step toward healing and acceptance.

## THE SCIENCE BEHIND TRAUMA: WHAT HAPPENS IN YOUR BRAIN

Understanding PTSD requires understanding the human brain, where trauma leaves its fingerprints. The amygdala, a small almond-shaped cluster of nuclei deep within the temporal lobes, plays a central role in processing fear. It acts as an alarm system, alerting us to danger, so when trauma occurs, the amygdala becomes hyperactive, interpreting even benign situations as threats.

This state of heightened alertness explains why someone with PTSD might find themselves startled by a sudden noise or panicked in a crowded room (Cleveland Clinic 2023). The hippocampus, meanwhile, is tasked with forming new memories and connecting them to emotions. In PTSD, hippocampus function is impaired, leading to difficulties in distinguishing past from present, resulting in vivid flashbacks and intrusive memories. Trauma alters brain chemistry, disrupting neural pathways and creating a cycle where fear and anxiety become constant companions (Anand and Dikhav 2012).

The physiological response to trauma is equally telling. When faced with a perceived threat, the body initiates the fight-or-flight response, releasing stress hormones like cortisol and norepinephrine. These hormones prepare the body to react swiftly to danger. In PTSD, though, this response becomes chronic, keeping the body in a constant state of readiness, even when there is no immediate threat. Over time, such prolonged exposure to stress hormones can lead to a variety of health issues, including heart problems, digestive disorders, and compromised immune function. This biological state of hyperarousal is both exhausting and debilitating, contributing to the fatigue and heightened anxiety commonly experienced by those with PTSD (McFarlane 2010).

Understanding these scientific principles provides insight into the everyday challenges faced by individuals with PTSD. Hypervigilance, for instance, is less a symptom than it is a manifestation of the brain's altered state. It explains why some individuals find it difficult to relax or feel safe, even in familiar environments. Anxiety, too, is rooted in these neurochemical changes, and it often leads to avoidance behaviors and social withdrawal. Recognizing the brain's role in these experiences can empower individuals to manage their symptoms more effectively. For example, knowing that the amygdala is overreacting can help one reframe their thoughts during a panic attack, reminding themselves that they're safe despite the alarm bells ringing in their mind. Granted, it's not that simple; you can't just turn off what your brain is doing because you know that, logically, it doesn't make sense. But it does help as a starting point.

For long-term solutions, there is hope in the concept of neuroplasticity—the brain's remarkable ability to adapt and rewire itself. This potential for change offers a pathway to recovery, especially through mindfulness practices, which can help calm the amygdala and reduce the intensity of the fear response. Mindfulness encourages present-moment awareness, which can help individuals step back from intrusive thoughts and focus on the here and now. Therapy, particularly trauma-focused approaches, can also promote healing by creating new neural pathways that counteract the effects of trauma. Through consistent practice and support, individuals can reshape their brain's response to stress, leading to a reduction in symptoms and improved quality of life (von Bernhardi et al. 2017).

While the brain's response to trauma is significant, it is not immutable. With the right tools and support, healing is both possible and attainable. The brain's capacity to heal and adapt is a testament to human resilience and an excellent guide for overcoming and adapting to PTSD.

## RECOGNIZING SYMPTOMS: THE SILENT IMPACTS ON DAILY LIFE

Living with PTSD often means dealing with a world filled with invisible barriers where ordinary tasks can trigger extraordinary challenges. For many, the most pervasive of these are intrusive thoughts and memories that interrupt daily activities—seemingly out of nowhere. These unwelcome reminders of past trauma can surface while doing the simplest chores, like folding laundry or making breakfast, turning everyday moments into stressful situations. If you're trying to focus on a conversation or a task at work, only to be pulled back into a memory that feels as vivid as the present, it's a painful disruption that can make even the most routine activities feel daunting.

Avoidance behaviors are another hallmark of PTSD, manifesting as a reluctance to engage with people or places associated with trauma —or sometimes even those that aren't. This can severely affect social interactions and relationships; you might withdraw from family gatherings, avoid crowded places, or isolate yourself from friends. The fear of encountering a trigger can lead to a shrinking world where the safety in solitude outweighs the risk of potential exposure. While these behaviors do protect you in the short term, they can also inadvertently deepen your feelings of loneliness and disconnect, creating a cycle that's hard to break.

Beyond these more apparent symptoms, PTSD often carries subtler emotional and cognitive challenges. Emotional numbness is a particularly insidious one, leaving you feeling detached from your surroundings and the people you love, unable to experience joy from things you've always leaned on for entertainment. This detachment can also make it difficult to experience connection, leading to strained relationships and a sense of alienation from one's own life. Coupled with this is the struggle to concentrate or remember details, which can impact personal and professional life alike in all sorts of ways. Misplacing keys or forgetting important dates may seem trivial, but when compounded by the weight of PTSD, they can contribute to a sense of inadequacy and frustration, turning the whole problem into a self-reinforcing downward spiral.

The workplace can also be a minefield of challenges for someone with PTSD. A constant pressure to perform, coupled with a fear of judgment or misunderstanding, can exacerbate your symptoms. Colleagues might notice mood swings or irritability, unaware of what you're dealing with underneath. Deadlines and meetings might trigger anxiety, leading you to procrastination or avoidance. At home, these same challenges might spill over, causing family issues as an inability to regulate emotions can lead to outbursts of anger or periods of withdrawal, leaving your loved ones feeling confused and hurt. As your relationships strain under the weight of these symptoms, you might feel increasing guilt and helplessness.

Sorting through these challenges requires self-assessment and awareness. By identifying personal symptom patterns, you can start to understand your triggers and responses; this self-awareness is the first step in seeking help and ultimately developing coping strategies. Self-reflection exercises, such as journaling about daily experiences and emotions, can provide valuable insights into your symptom patterns, as these exercises encourage a deeper understanding of one's emotional environment, offering a clearer picture of when and why you're having certain reactions.

Knowing when to seek professional support is equally important because you shouldn't expect yourself to do this all on your own. Professional guidance can offer tailored strategies to manage your symptoms and improve your quality of life. If your symptoms persistently interfere with daily functioning or relationships, it may be time to reach out for help. Therapy can provide a safe space to explore these challenges and develop effective coping mechanisms, allowing you to begin to reclaim your life, step by step.

## INTERSECTIONAL INSIGHTS: HOW CULTURE AND GENDER SHAPE PTSD

The experience of PTSD is not a monolith; it is heavily shaped by culture, which influences how individuals perceive and manage their symptoms. In many cultures, mental health is often seen as a weakness or a spiritual failing, leading people who suffer from mental health issues to feel stigmatized and to endure their struggles in silence, fearing judgment or ostracization. In communities where stoicism is valued, expressing vulnerability may be discouraged, leading you to internalize your issues. Cultural stigmas can thus impede access to care, as you might hesitate to seek help or acknowledge your symptoms, viewing them as personal failures rather than medical conditions.

The way PTSD manifests can also differ across cultural lines. In some cultures, emotional expression is generally considered more acceptable, leading to open displays of distress—but in other cultures, which prioritize emotional restraint, the expressions of PTSD might be more somatic, such as with physical pain or fatigue. Understanding these differences is extremely important for providing effective support and treatment. You have to think about cultural context when diagnosing and treating PTSD, as what may be a clear symptom in one culture could be something entirely different in another.

Gender also plays an important role in shaping the PTSD experience. Women, for example, are more likely to experience gender-based trauma such as domestic violence or sexual assault; statistics indicate roughly one in three women worldwide suffer either physical or sexual violence (or both) during their lifetime (World Health Organization 2024). This can, in turn, lead to distinct manifestations of PTSD. Societal expectations often dictate that women remain composed and nurturing, even in the face of trauma, which can lead to feelings of isolation and shame when they struggle internally. It isn't helped by the fact police forces can sometimes minimize or outright dismiss charges of sexual assault even in the 5 percent of cases that actually get reported (Murphy-Oikonen et al. 2020).

Men, on the other hand, may face different challenges. Societal norms often pressure men to suppress their emotions, as vulnerability is equated with weakness. This can result in underreporting of symptoms and reluctance to seek therapy as men grapple with the fear of being perceived as less masculine. Though the numbers are on the rise, studies have shown that a significantly higher percentage of women seek therapeutic help as compared to men (Terlizzi and Schiller 2022).

Incorporating voices from diverse backgrounds can illuminate the varied experiences of those who suffer from PTSD. Let's say there's a young mother from a conservative community whose PTSD stems from years of domestic abuse. Seeking help for her might mean defying entrenched social norms, highlighting the intersection of cultural and gender influences. Similarly, we might talk about a refugee who, after fleeing conflict, finds himself in a new country that does not recognize his trauma as legitimate because it doesn't fit the local narrative of mental health. Stories like these emphasize the need for an intersectional approach to understanding PTSD, one that acknowledges both cultural and gender issues.

To effectively address these complexities, culturally sensitive approaches to treatment are necessary. This means therapists must adapt their techniques to accommodate cultural differences, perhaps by integrating traditional healing practices with conventional therapy. Incorporating community-based interventions that match cultural values can encourage participation. Finding culturally competent therapists who understand the various cultural nuances of PTSD can also make a significant difference. This involves therapists who are both aware of cultural backgrounds and actively incorporate this understanding into their practice, creating a safe space for clients to express themselves without fear of judgment.

Ultimately, recognizing the intersectionality of culture and gender in PTSD experiences allows for more personalized, effective care. By acknowledging these diverse narratives, we create a more inclusive understanding of PTSD that respects the unique challenges each individual faces. This approach leads to better support and empowers individuals to seek help that aligns with their cultural and personal identity.

## THE THERAPEUTIC ALLIANCE: FINDING THE RIGHT SUPPORT

The connection between therapist and client—known as the therapeutic alliance—is the bedrock of effective therapy. This bond isn't simply a cordial relationship but involves creating a space where trust flourishes and healing becomes possible. A strong therapeutic alliance is built on mutual respect, empathy, and understanding, allowing individuals to explore their vulnerabilities without fear of judgment. The key elements of this alliance include a shared agreement on therapy goals, collaboration on tasks, and the development of an emotional bond, ultimately creating a safe environment amidst the often chaotic psychological experience of PTSD.

If this sounds familiar to you, it's important to choose the right therapist to establish this alliance. Therapists with experience in trauma-focused therapies understand the nuances of PTSD and can offer approaches tailored to your trauma, but personal compatibility is still the single most important factor in whether your therapy will have a good outcome. The therapist's communication style, empathy, and ability to create a comfortable space all matter, so ask potential therapists about their experience with PTSD, their therapeutic approach, and how they handle setbacks. Think about how you feel during initial interactions—do you feel heard and understood? A lot of this really does come down to vibes, so don't be afraid to go with your instincts.

Various therapeutic approaches, meanwhile, offer different paths to healing PTSD. Cognitive-behavioral therapy (CBT) is one of the most effective methods, focusing on identifying and changing negative thought patterns and behaviors. CBT empowers individuals to regain control over their thoughts and emotions, increasing their resilience and reducing their symptoms (Corliss 2024). Eye Movement Desensitization and Reprocessing (EMDR) is another powerful tool, using guided eye movements to process traumatic memories and soften their emotional impact—an approach that can be particularly beneficial for those who struggle with intrusive memories (American Psychological Association 2023). While these therapies are widely recognized, some people also find respite through alternative therapies such as art therapy or somatic experiencing. These methods engage the mind and body, allowing for expression and healing beyond words.

Therapy is not without its challenges, and setbacks are a natural part of the process. It's important to manage your expectations in order to maintain your motivation. Progress may be slow, and at times, it might feel as if you're treading water, but you should always remember that healing is not linear. Effective communication with your therapist can help you deal with these challenges, so be open about your feelings and concerns. If a particular approach doesn't seem to be working, discuss alternatives. Therapy is a collaborative process, and your input is valuable in shaping the direction and focus of sessions.

In moments of doubt or frustration, remember the purpose of therapy: to support and guide you through dealing with PTSD. A strong therapeutic alliance offers a refuge where you can explore your experiences and emotions, providing you with the tools to face your challenges, to find strength in vulnerability, and to continue moving forward. Therapy is ultimately about reclaiming your life one step at a time.

## DEALING WITH THE MENTAL HEALTH SYSTEM: YOUR ESSENTIAL GUIDE

Unfortunately, working with the mental health system can often feel like stepping into a maze, especially when you're already overwhelmed. You have to deal with the divide between public and private services, as each has its own set of protocols and resources. Public mental health services, funded by government programs in certain countries, aim to provide accessible care to all, often at a lower cost. However, these services can be stretched thin, resulting in longer wait times and limited availability. Private services, on the other hand, offer more immediate access and specialized care but at a higher price, which can be a barrier for many. It's up to you which route you decide to take.

Within this framework, a variety of professionals serve important roles. Psychiatrists, who are medical doctors, can prescribe medication and manage complex conditions. Psychologists, meanwhile, provide therapy and conduct assessments, while social workers can help deal with social services and offer counseling. Each professional brings unique expertise, and knowing who does what can streamline your search for the right support.

Finding and utilizing mental health resources requires a proactive approach (which can often feel like one of the biggest barriers to entry). Local services can often be found through community health centers or online directories, and you should look for reviews and recommendations to gauge the quality of care and whether the type of service is right for you. In the United States, it's also important to understand your insurance coverage; some plans may cover only certain types of therapy or specific providers, so check the details carefully. If finances are a concern—and they could well be, as therapy often isn't cheap—investigate sliding scale options or community programs that offer reduced fees. The path to care is not always straightforward, and walking it requires persistence and self-advocacy.

It's true that barriers to accessing care are common, but they're not insurmountable. Long wait times can be discouraging, but there are ways to mitigate them, such as joining support groups or engaging in self-help strategies. These may be interim measures, but they can still provide relief and support. Self-advocacy is key, too; don't hesitate to follow up on referrals or ask for cancellations to expedite appointments—you might feel like you're being a pest, but you have every right to seek care. Additionally, if a particular resource isn't available in your area, explore telehealth options, which have expanded access to care significantly in recent years. There are more resources out there than you might think, from online therapy platforms to mental health apps, all of which can potentially supplement traditional care.

Community and peer support are invaluable as you work through these issues. Connecting with others who share similar experiences can offer comfort and understanding that professional care alone may not provide. Support groups, whether in person or online, create spaces where you can share your story without fear of judgment. Community resources, such as local nonprofits or advocacy groups, often offer workshops and events that promote mental health awareness and provide additional layers of support.

As you deal with this complex system, remember that reaching out is a sign of strength, not weakness. When you reach out, you're acknowledging your needs and showing a commitment to your well-being, and that's something to be celebrated. The path may be winding, but every step forward is a testament to your resilience. Embrace the connections you build along the way, and let them fortify you. Community, both professional and personal, is a powerful ally in your quest for healing. As you continue, hold onto the knowledge that you are not alone, and that support is within reach.

CHAPTER 2

# BUILDING A FOUNDATION OF SELF-COMPASSION

Let's say you're watching a child learn to ride a bike. They wobble, fall, and scrape their knees. Instinctively, you're likely to rush to their side, offering comforting words and a gentle hand. You'll want to reassure them that it's okay to fall, that learning takes time, and that they're brave for trying! Given that you're willing to extend kindness to others ... why don't you offer the same level of compassion to yourself when you stumble? That's where self-compassion comes into play.

## WHAT IS SELF-COMPASSION?

Self-compassion is the practice of treating yourself with the same kindness and understanding you'd extend to a child or a dear friend. Supporting others is a natural human tendency, but supporting yourself sometimes takes some effort. The judgmental voices in your head can and should become a gentle, supportive dialogue if you want your own brain to aid in trauma recovery.

At its core, self-compassion consists of three components, as described by Professor Kristin Neff: self-kindness, common humanity, and mindfulness. Self-kindness involves being gentle with yourself in moments of pain or failure rather than judging yourself with undue harshness. Common humanity recognizes that suffering and personal inadequacy are part of the shared human experience—something we all go through rather than something that isolates us. Mindfulness requires that we hold our painful thoughts and feelings in balanced awareness rather than over-identifying with them. Each component works in tandem to create a robust framework for emotional resilience and healing (Harrison 2022).

It's important to distinguish self-compassion from self-pity and self-indulgence. Self-pity involves wallowing in your own problems, forgetting that other people have similar struggles. Self-indulgence, on the other hand, might mean letting yourself off the hook too easily, thus avoiding your responsibilities. True self-compassion, meanwhile, is an active process of caring for yourself responsibly and honestly, maintaining a balance between acknowledging your challenges and encouraging your growth.

The benefits of self-compassion in trauma recovery are significant. By practicing self-compassion, you can significantly reduce levels of anxiety and depression and encourage emotional stability and resilience, allowing you to face challenges with a calm and balanced mindset. When you treat yourself with kindness, your perspective shifts; setbacks become opportunities for learning rather than failures to be ashamed of. This shift can lead to greater emotional stability as you learn to regulate your emotions with understanding and patience.

Let's say you make a mistake at work that costs your team time. Your initial reaction might be to criticize yourself harshly, replaying the error repeatedly in your mind. Self-compassion, though, would invite you to acknowledge your mistake, understand it in the context of being human, and decide on a constructive path forward. This approach ultimately empowers you to make amends without the weight of self-condemnation, avoiding the trap of allowing one mistake to compound another. Similarly, during recovery from trauma, you're going to see some setbacks—it's just a natural part of the process. Practicing patience with yourself when you stumble develops your resilience, allowing you to continue moving forward without being completely derailed by temporary stumbles.

So, how do you make sure to embrace self-compassion as a daily practice? Simple: change your mindset to one that deliberately encourages self-kindness. This involves integrating affirmations and mantras into your routine; phrases like "I am enough just as I am" or "I choose to be kind to myself today" can serve as powerful reminders of your commitment to self-compassion. Additionally, visualization exercises, where you picture a supportive inner dialogue, can help create a nurturing mental environment. Picture a trusted friend or mentor speaking to you with kindness and encouragement, guiding you through difficult moments.

### *Reflective Exercise: Cultivating Self-Compassion*

Take a moment to reflect on a recent challenge. Write down the judgmental thoughts you had about yourself. Now, reframe those thoughts with compassion; what would a supportive friend say? Write down these compassionate responses and read them aloud. Notice how this shift in perspective feels in your body and mind.

By practicing self-compassion in your daily life, you open the door to a more gentle and understanding relationship with yourself. This foundation supports your healing and strengthens your capacity to deal with life's struggles with grace and resilience.

## OVERCOMING SELF-CRITICISM: YOUR INNER DIALOGUE

The roots of self-criticism often run deep, tracing back to childhood experiences and the societal pressures that shape our sense of self-worth. As children, we absorb the attitudes and beliefs of those around us, especially authority figures like parents and teachers. If you were criticized or held to impossibly high standards, you might have internalized those voices, carrying them into adulthood as your own. Society compounds this by bombarding us with images and messages of perfection. These external voices then become internalized scripts, replaying in your mind, telling you that you must do better, be better, and not show weakness.

Trauma, meanwhile, can intensify this internal dialogue, casting a long shadow over your perception of self. When you've experienced trauma, these voices often grow louder, feeding on vulnerability and inadequacy trauma might have drilled into you. It can feel like the trauma opened the door for self-doubt to take a more prominent place in your psyche, amplifying the negative self-talk until it feels like an unending loop.

This cycle of negative self-talk can be incredibly damaging, ultimately undermining your efforts to heal and recover. Think about the common self-defeating thoughts that arise in the aftermath of trauma: "I'm broken," "I should have handled it better," or "I don't deserve happiness." These thoughts are deeply unkind to yourself, sure, but they also create a barrier to recovery by reinforcing feelings of shame and inadequacy. When you constantly criticize yourself, it can lead to a downward spiral, where each mistake, each perceived failure, becomes evidence of your unworthiness. This cycle erodes your mental health, contributing to anxiety, depression, and a pervasive sense of hopelessness. With each turn of this cycle, your emotional well-being takes a hit, making it harder to see a path forward.

To counter self-criticism, it's important to develop strategies that turn these negative dialogues into supportive ones in order to break that cycle. Start with cognitive restructuring exercises, which are designed to challenge and reframe negative thoughts. When a difficult thought arises, pause and ask yourself: Is this thought true? What evidence do I have to support it? Often, you'll find that these thoughts are based on assumptions rather than facts, and you can replace them with more balanced, compassionate perspectives. If you catch yourself thinking, "I'm such a failure," you might reframe it as, "I made a mistake, but that doesn't define me." This shift in perspective alleviates the heavy burden of self-criticism without ignoring your mistake entirely, allowing you to view situations with greater clarity and kindness.

Practicing self-compassionate responses in moments of self-doubt is another effective approach. When you notice self-doubt creeping in, treat yourself as you would a close friend. Remind yourself that everyone makes mistakes and that these experiences are opportunities for learning and growth. This practice can feel foreign at first, especially if you're accustomed to harsh self-judgment, but over time, it can create a more nurturing internal environment. It might take time, but keep at it, and eventually, you'll get there.

Supportive inner dialogue exercises can further help cultivate a nurturing inner monologue. Role-playing exercises for positive self-talk are particularly useful; think of yourself as an actor rehearsing lines for a play, but instead of reciting someone else's words, you're creating affirmations and supportive statements for yourself. Practice these lines daily, allowing them to become a natural part of your thought process. Additionally, journaling can be a powerful tool for identifying and altering judgmental thoughts using prompts like "What would I say to a friend in my situation?" or "How can I reframe this thought more positively?" Regular journaling helps uncover patterns of self-criticism and provides a space to consciously shift toward a more compassionate dialogue.

***Reflection Section: Rewriting Your Inner Script***

Take a moment to think about a recurring self-critical thought. Write it down and then challenge it by asking, "Is this thought helping or harming me?" Next, rewrite the thought in a way that is supportive and encouraging, as if you were speaking to a loved one. Reflect on how this new perspective feels and how it might influence your day-to-day life.

These practices aren't about ignoring your challenges or sugar-coating reality. Instead, they're about acknowledging your struggles while recognizing your strengths and potential for growth. By changing your inner dialogue, you create a foundation of compassion that supports you throughout your healing.

## PRACTICAL EXERCISES FOR DAILY SELF-COMPASSION

One important thing to remember is that integrating self-compassion into your daily life doesn't have to be complicated. One simple practice is the "self-compassion break," designed for those moments when stress and self-doubt creep in. When you notice your emotional temperature rising, pause and place a hand over your heart. Take a deep breath and silently acknowledge your feelings, saying, "This is a moment of suffering. Suffering is a part of life." Then, gently remind yourself, "May I be kind to myself." This small act can shift your mindset from criticism to compassion, allowing you to pause and reset emotionally.

Daily gratitude journaling is another powerful tool. Each day, take a few moments to jot down things you appreciate about yourself, whether it's your resilience in facing challenges or your ability to bring a smile to someone else's face. These small acknowledgments can build a foundation of self-appreciation, boosting your self-worth over time. It's important to understand that small steps are still steps, and ultimately, they add up to something larger.

Ritualizing these practices can help them become a natural part of your routine. Maybe start your morning with a self-reflection ritual: As you drink your coffee or tea, take a moment to think about the day ahead. Set an intention for how you wish to treat yourself and others with kindness. In the evening, revisit this intention, thinking about how you honored it and where you can improve. Create a self-compassionate morning affirmation routine by choosing a few affirmations that work for you personally. Repeat them to yourself as you prepare for the day. Phrases like "I am worthy of love and respect" or "I embrace my flaws and strengths" can reinforce a positive mindset, setting a tone of self-love from the moment you wake up.

Physical self-care is equally important in nurturing self-compassion, too. Gentle yoga and stretching are acts of kindness to your body, helping release tension and promote relaxation. These practices encourage you to listen to your body's needs and respond with care. As you move, focus on your breathing and how your body feels, allowing yourself to be fully present. Preparing nourishing meals can also be a form of self-care. As you cook, engage your senses—notice the colors of vegetables, the sound of sizzling, and the aroma of spices. Approach each meal with gratitude for the nourishment it provides, savoring each bite as an act of self-love and taking pride in what you've created.

Mindful self-compassion meditations can also help encourage a sense of inner peace and acceptance. Guided loving-kindness meditation focused on the self involves sitting quietly and repeating phrases like "May I be happy, may I be healthy, may I be safe" with sincerity and intention. This meditation nurtures a gentle, caring relationship with yourself. Visualizations can further boost this practice: maybe picture a warm, golden light enveloping you, representing self-love and acceptance. Allow this light to fill you with warmth and comfort, dissolving tension and self-doubt. These meditative practices serve to both provide moments of calm and cultivate a lasting sense of compassion that grows stronger with each session. Self-compassion really is like any other muscle, in that it gets stronger the more you work on it.

## MINDFULNESS AND SELF-ACCEPTANCE: A DUAL APPROACH

In the midst of life's chaos, mindfulness offers a haven of presence and acceptance. Mindfulness involves cultivating a non-judgmental awareness of your thoughts and feelings, allowing them to exist without the need to change or suppress them. This practice encourages you to observe your inner world without attachment, granting you a sense of peace and clarity. At its heart, mindfulness revolves around three principles: presence, acceptance, and non-judgment. Presence invites you to live in the moment, fully engaged with your surroundings. Acceptance encourages you to embrace your experiences—regardless of their nature—without resistance. Non-judgment involves observing your thoughts and emotions without labeling them as good or bad. Together, these principles create a framework for self-awareness and emotional balance, which is exactly what you need if you're healing from trauma.

The synergy between mindfulness and self-compassion lies in their mutual reinforcement. When you are mindful, you approach your experiences with openness and curiosity, providing a space to develop self-compassion. In trauma recovery, this combination is particularly powerful, as mindfulness helps you step back from the autopilot reactions trauma can often trigger, instead creating a pause where self-compassion can intervene. Let's say someone with PTSD experiences a flashback. Mindfulness allows them to recognize the flashback as a momentary occurrence rather than a permanent reality. In that space, self-compassion can offer comfort and reassurance, reminding them of their strength and resilience. This interplay between mindfulness and self-compassion can change the way you engage with your trauma, shifting from a place of struggle to one of healing.

Mindfulness exercises can also be invaluable in cultivating self-acceptance. One effective method is the body scan meditation, which guides you through a focused awareness of each part of your body. As you direct attention to different areas, you observe your sensations without judgment, helping create a sense of connection and acceptance. This practice can reveal how emotions manifest physically, offering insights into your mind-body relationship. Mindful breathing exercises are another tool to cultivate calm and presence: By focusing on the rhythm of your breath, you ground yourself in the present moment, easing your anxiety and replacing it with clarity. These exercises encourage you to accept your experiences as they are without the need to fix or change them.

Creating a balanced routine that integrates mindfulness and self-compassion takes a little bit of forethought, starting with developing a personal mindfulness practice schedule that matches up with your lifestyle. Maybe dedicate a few minutes each morning or evening to mindfulness exercises, allowing them to become a regular part of your daily rhythm. This consistency reinforces the habit, making mindfulness a natural response to life's challenges. Just like with gratitude and affirmations, combining mindfulness with journaling can help you deepen your self-reflection. After a mindfulness session, take a moment to jot down your observations and insights; this can encourage a dialogue between your mind and emotions, boosting your self-awareness and self-acceptance. It can also reveal patterns and triggers, offering valuable guidance on your healing path.

As you integrate these practices, acknowledge that where you're headed isn't a straightforward line. Healing from trauma is a process that requires patience and kindness toward yourself; mindfulness and self-compassion are not quick fixes but lifelong companions, offering solace and strength in moments of uncertainty. They invite you to be present with your experiences, to accept yourself as you are, and to cultivate a gentle resilience that carries you forward.

## JOURNALING FOR HEALING: WRITING YOUR PATH TO RECOVERY

I've mentioned journaling a couple of times, but it bears going into a little more detail. Journaling can offer a unique avenue for emotional processing, a quiet space where thoughts and feelings can unfold without judgment. The act of writing can unearth your subconscious thoughts, bringing hidden emotions to the surface and allowing you to deal with them. Writing can help you explore and articulate what you might not readily express aloud by bypassing the filters we sometimes unconsciously set up for ourselves. It can be one of the best ways to gain insight into your inner world, tracing patterns and uncovering things that might otherwise elude you. Journaling is ultimately a mirror, reflecting your unfiltered self back at you.

There are specific techniques that can encourage self-compassion and growth with journaling, too. One such exercise is writing a "Letter to Your Future Self," focusing on hope and potential. In this exercise, picture yourself five or ten years down the road. What would you like to tell this future self? What dreams or aspirations do you hope they've achieved? This exercise both reinforces a sense of direction and instills a belief in your capacity to grow and heal.

A "Gratitude Journal" can be another powerful technique. Here, the focus is on recognizing your personal strengths and achievements. Each entry provides an opportunity to celebrate small victories, reinforcing a positive self-image and cultivating a mindset of appreciation. This nurtures a sense of fulfillment, grounding you in the present while acknowledging the progress you've already made.

Storytelling through journaling plays an important role in recovery. By structuring your personal narratives, you gain perspective and understanding, allowing you to step back from your experiences and view them as stories with a beginning, middle, and end. It provides a framework for making sense of past events—taking chaos and converting it into coherence. Reflective writing on past experiences invites healing by encouraging introspection, allowing you to confront your trauma, process it, and ultimately reshape your own narrative. This act of storytelling also imbues your experiences with meaning, turning them from random occurrences into chapters of a larger, more comprehensible story.

Creating a consistent journaling routine boosts the benefits of this practice. Dedicate a specific time each day to write, whether in the quiet of the morning or the stillness of the night, allowing consistency to reinforce the habit and provide a steady touchpoint for reflection. Developing a comfortable and inspiring writing space can further enrich this experience, so choose a spot that feels safe and inviting—maybe near a window with natural light or surrounded by calming elements like plants or gentle music. Let this space be a sanctuary where you can freely express your thoughts and emotions without fear of intrusion—this is your space and no one else's.

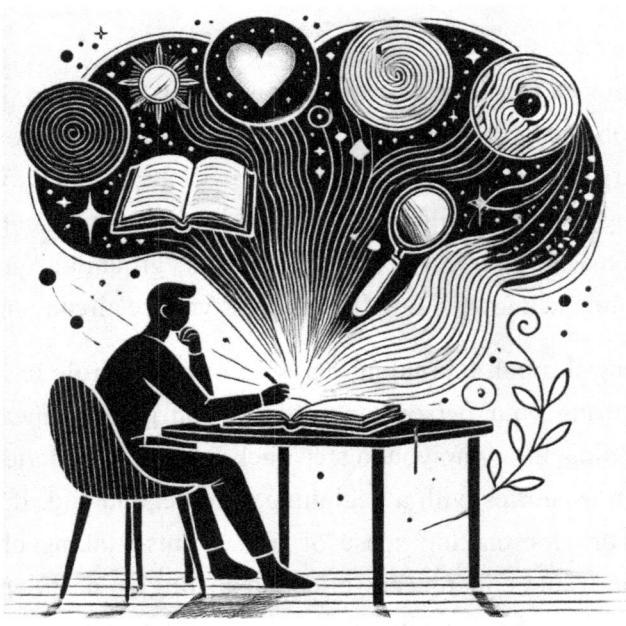

As you establish this routine, allow yourself the freedom to explore without constraint. Your journal is a private space, a haven where you can write without the pressure of external validation. Embrace the process as an opportunity for growth and self-discovery, trusting that each entry, no matter how seemingly insignificant, contributes to your healing.

## CREATING A SAFE SPACE: YOUR SANCTUARY FOR GROWTH

About that private space: you need to develop it to your own specifications. This space is your sanctuary, a personal refuge that nurtures both your mind and your spirit. Having a quiet corner is nice, but ultimately, it's more important to create an environment that supports emotional healing and encourages self-discovery. In this space, you can reflect without distraction, allowing your thoughts and emotions to surface in a safe and controlled manner, free from triggers that can bring them up when you're not expecting them. Whether it's a nook in your home or a mental retreat you construct in your mind, this sanctuary is hugely important for personal growth. It's where you can pause, breathe, and explore your inner mindscape without fear or judgment.

Designing your safe space requires intention and care. If you're dealing with a physical space, it can be a good idea to select colors that soothe and calm, such as soft blues or gentle greens, as these hues can create a serene atmosphere, promoting relaxation and peace. The decor matters a lot here, and you should put thought into it, choosing items that bring you comfort and joy. Maybe these include a favorite painting, a plush chair, or a soft blanket—whatever you pick, it should be elements designed to invite you to settle in and unwind. Incorporating natural elements like plants can also improve the ambiance, bringing a touch of the outdoors inside. Plants really do have health benefits, as the presence of greenery has actually been shown to reduce stress and improve mental clarity (Haupt 2023). Thoughtful lighting matters, too, so opt for soft, warm lights that create a cozy glow, avoiding harsh, bright lights that can disrupt a tranquil mood.

Once your sanctuary is set, it becomes the perfect setting for meditation or yoga sessions (among other things). Quietly stretching your body in a space that feels comforting and private allows you to let go of stress and reconnect with your breath. You could also use this space to engage in creative expression through art or music and allow yourself to paint, draw, play an instrument, or simply listen to your favorite tunes. Your goal here isn't to produce something perfect; you just want to let your creativity flow and find joy in the process. Your sanctuary is a judgment-free zone where you can explore what truly makes you feel alive and connected.

The emotional significance of your safe space is the single most important part of the process. It's a retreat where you can practice self-compassion and introspection—components you can't forego in the healing process. Use this space for reflection and self-care rituals that rejuvenate your spirit, whatever those may be. Perhaps it's reading a book that inspires you or writing in a journal that captures your thoughts and dreams, but whatever works for you is what you need to do. Establishing firm boundaries around this space is necessary for maintaining its sanctity, so let it be known that this is your time and place for solitude and self-care, free from external demands. Protect this sanctuary fiercely, as it is where your most authentic self can emerge and thrive.

As you cultivate this safe haven, remember that it exists as both a physical and emotional space. This haven is present wherever you feel secure and at peace, even if it's simply within your mind. This sanctuary is a major part of your healing, as it offers a respite from the chaos of the outside world. Here, in the quiet and stillness, you can truly listen to yourself, explore your desires, and nurture the parts of you that need love and attention.

Creating this sanctuary ultimately serves to lay the groundwork for deeper self-exploration and healing. As you continue to build upon this foundation, always bear in mind the principles of self-compassion and mindfulness. Your sanctuary will be a steadfast ally, supporting you as you deal with your emotions and experiences.

CHAPTER 3

# DEALING WITH EMOTIONAL TURBULENCE

Dealing with roiling, frequently conflicting emotions can feel daunting, especially when you're confronted with intense waves of fear, anger, or sadness. These reactions often seem to come out of nowhere, crashing into your daily life with unexpected force. They can come from anywhere - a phone call, a news report, a certain smell in the air, leaving you with a nasty emotional surprise that sets off one of your triggers and ruins your entire day. This is the nature of emotional triggers—they are powerful reminders of past trauma lurking beneath the surface, ready to emerge at a moment's notice.

## HOW TO COPE WITH TRIGGERS

Understanding and managing these triggers is how you reclaim control over your emotional world. You'll need to start by identifying and categorizing your personal triggers; these are often specific stimuli—certain sounds, smells, places, or even people—that provoke strong emotional responses. Journaling is an excellent tool to help uncover patterns in these reactions if you're not already sure what they are. Keep a detailed record of your emotional responses throughout the day, noting the context, the trigger, and how you felt both physically and mentally while it was happening. Over time, you'll start to see patterns emerge, revealing the triggers that impact you most and allowing you to anticipate and prepare for them.

The link between these triggers and past trauma is often significant, and understanding this connection can help a lot with emotional management. Let's say there's a soldier who finds the sound of fireworks deeply unsettling. Clearly, it's not the fireworks themselves but the association with gunfire and chaos that evokes such a visceral reaction. Similarly, a survivor of domestic violence might find a particular cologne triggering if it was worn by their abuser. Reflecting on past experiences can help you identify where your own triggers came from, providing clarity in helping you differentiate between the past and the present and reminding you that the danger is no longer real.

Developing a personalized trigger map can further aid in managing your emotional responses. This involves visually organizing your triggers to better understand and manage them with a chart or diagram mapping out each trigger and its associated emotional response. Include notes on the intensity and frequency of each reaction. This visual representation can serve as a valuable reference, helping you see the connections and patterns more clearly. There are various ways to create this map, from simple lists to more complex diagrams; ultimately, just use whatever works best for you.

**How to Use the Trigger Map:**

1. **Identify triggers**: Write down situations, sounds, smells, or events that provoke a strong emotional or physical reaction.
2. **Track emotional responses**: Note how you feel when exposed to each trigger (e.g., fear, anger, sadness).
3. **Record physical responses**: Include any bodily reactions (e.g., racing heart, shaking, nausea).
4. **Rate intensity**: Use a 1-10 scale to quantify how intense the reaction feels.
5. **Log frequency**: Note how often the trigger occurs.
6. **Look for patterns**: Use the notes section to identify recurring themes or insights.

This trigger map can help you recognize connections between triggers and reactions, enabling you to develop coping strategies tailored to your unique needs. You can also bring this map to a therapist to collaborate on further interventions.

Now that you know what your triggers are, you can implement proactive strategies to manage them. One approach is planning to avoid environments or situations that you know will provoke a strong reaction; if crowded places make you anxious, you might want to visit during off-peak hours or use earplugs to minimize noise. But avoidance isn't always possible or even advisable, so developing coping mechanisms can help minimize the impact when you do encounter a trigger. Techniques such as deep breathing, visualization, or positive affirmations can help bring you back to yourself in these moments, grounding you and reminding you of your safety, in turn allowing you to regain control over your emotions.

## Creating Your Trigger Map

Take a moment to sit down with a pen and paper. List your known triggers, and next to each one, jot down the emotions and physical sensations they provoke. Now, try to trace each trigger back to its origin—what past event or experience might it be linked to? Create a visual representation of these connections. This exercise can help clarify your triggers and empower you with the knowledge to manage them more effectively.

As you explore these strategies, remember that emotional triggers are not your enemy; they're signals from your mind, calling attention to areas that require healing. By understanding and managing them, you're taking a significant step toward emotional balance and peace.

Here is an example of a trigger map. This example uses a table format for simplicity, but you can adapt it into a diagram or chart.

| Trigger | Emotional Response | Physical Response | Intensity (1-10) |
|---|---|---|---|
| Loud sudden noises | Panic, fear | Heart racing, sweating | 9 |
| Crowded spaces | Anxiety, irritability | Shallow breathing, restlessness | 7 |
| Certain smells (e.g., smoke) | Flashbacks, sadness | Nausea, trembling | 8 |
| Arguments or raised voices | Anger, sadness | Muscle tension, shaking | 6 |
| Specific dates/events | Depression, grief | Lethargy, loss of appetite | 10 |

**Trigger Map Example**

*Please see the download link at the end of the book for your own personal Trigger Map.*

## GROUNDING TECHNIQUES: STAYING PRESENT IN THE NOW

When you're dealing with a lot of anxiety and distress, grounding techniques can serve as a lifeline, anchoring you firmly in the present moment. These techniques are extremely important in breaking the cycle of overwhelming emotions that PTSD can set off. When anxiety grips you, it often pulls you away from reality, plunging you into formless yet all-consuming fear and panic. Grounding acts as a stabilizer, providing a point of reference in the here and now, allowing you to regain control over your thoughts and emotions. By focusing on the immediate environment, you can interrupt the spiraling thoughts that fuel anxiety, restoring a sense of calm and focus. This practice will also sharpen your concentration, helping you work through daily challenges more easily.

There are a variety of grounding exercises you might integrate into your daily life, each offering simple yet effective ways to maintain presence and stability. The "5-4-3-2-1" sensory exercise is a powerful tool for immediate grounding. It involves identifying five things you can see, four things you can touch, three things you can hear, two things you can smell, and one thing you can taste. This exercise engages each of your senses, drawing your attention away from distressing thoughts and back to the physical world (Smith 2018).

An example of grounding exercises that you can track:

| Step | Examples | Your Input |
|---|---|---|
| 5 Things You Can See | e.g., A chair, the sky, a plant, your hands, a book | |
| 4 Things You Can Touch | e.g., The fabric of your shirt, the table, your hair, the ground | |
| 3 Things You Can Hear | e.g., Birds chirping, a clock ticking, distant traffic | |
| 2 Things You Can Smell | e.g., Freshly brewed coffee, a candle, a flower | |
| 1 Thing You Can Taste | e.g., Gum, a sip of water, the lingering taste of food | |

*A blank chart for your own 5-4-3-2-1 exercises is available through the downloadable workbook at the and of the book.*

Physical grounding through touch is another method that you can utilize anywhere as long as you have the object with you. Holding a comforting item, such as a smooth stone or a piece of fabric, can provide tactile reassurance, anchoring you in the present. You can also try placing your hands in water or picking up a piece of ice, both tactile sensations that can bring you back to the present moment. Mental grounding, on the other hand, involves focusing on factual details of your environment, such as the color of the walls or the number of windows in a room. This focus on concrete, observable elements helps redirect your mind from the abstract realm of anxiety to the tangible reality around you (Raypole 2024).

Incorporating grounding techniques into your daily routine is how you get them to be effective, with regular practice making them second nature when you need them most. Set reminders on your phone or place notes around your home to prompt these exercises throughout the day. You might also think about creating a personal checklist of preferred grounding methods that can serve as a quick reference, guiding you to the techniques that work best for you. Whether it's taking a few moments to engage in the 5-4-3-2-1 exercise or holding your favorite tactile object, these small acts of self-care can make a significant difference in your emotional well-being.

Grounding becomes particularly valuable during stressful situations, where anxiety tends to peak, and practicing grounding before, during, and after anticipated stressors can help manage your emotional responses. If you know that a specific event or encounter is likely to trigger anxiety, engage in a grounding exercise beforehand to calm your nerves. During the event, use grounding techniques to maintain presence and composure, and afterward, use them as a means of unwinding to process the experience. You might also combine grounding with other calming strategies, such as deep breathing or affirmations—both of which we'll cover in more detail shortly—to make them even more effective. Deep breathing helps regulate your body's stress response, while grounding keeps you connected to the present, creating a synergistic effect that helps calm your body and mind down.

Remember that these grounding techniques are tools for empowerment. They offer a way to deal with anxiety and distress, providing a steady anchor point amidst what can feel like emotional chaos. With practice and persistence, grounding can become an integral part of your coping arsenal, supporting you in finding peace and presence in every moment.

## MANAGING FLASHBACKS: TECHNIQUES FOR IMMEDIATE RELIEF

Flashbacks are a formidable obstacle with PTSD, transporting you back to the intense emotions and chaos of a traumatic event. Reliving your feelings might not involve actual visual imagery, but it can also be a full sensory experience involving vivid sights or scenes that play out in front of you as if they're happening all over again. You can be in a familiar setting like your living room when something as innocuous as a scent or a sound hurls you back to a moment filled with fear or helplessness. Unsurprisingly, these experiences can do quite a bit to disrupt your day, making the ordinary feel insurmountable and leaving you feeling vulnerable and disoriented.

During these episodes, you have to find a way to regain control in order to find your way back to the present. One effective strategy is deep breathing, which helps regulate your nervous system, slow your heart rate, and calm your mind. Inhale deeply through your nose, hold for a moment, and exhale slowly through your mouth. This deliberate focus on your breath can act as an anchor, pulling you back from the turmoil of a flashback. Repeating affirmations like "I am safe now" or "This moment is not the same as the past" reinforces your current reality, providing a reassuring counterbalance to the intensity of a flashback. It's important that you don't feel like a failure if doing this doesn't work immediately; it takes practice, and that's okay.

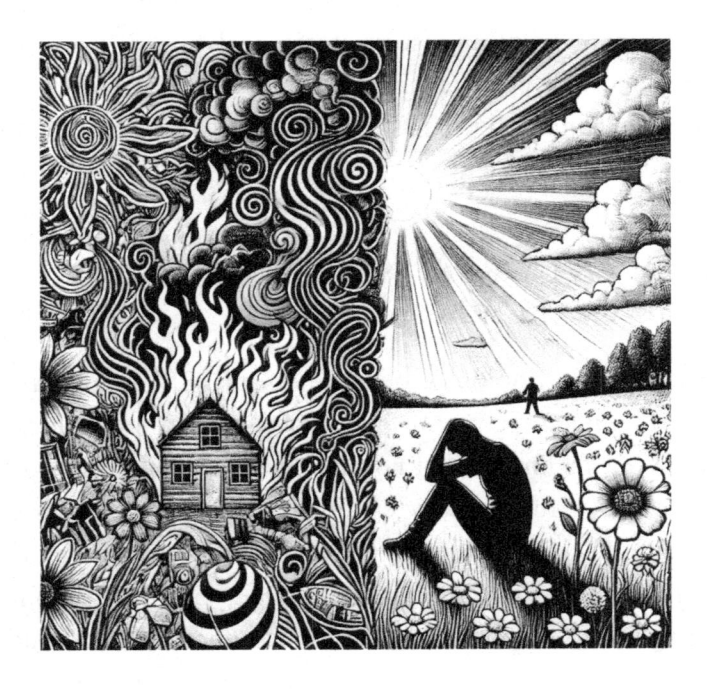

After the immediate distress of a flashback subsides, it's important to process and recover from what you've just dealt with. Journaling can help here, too, just like it does when figuring out your triggers. Write about the experience of the flashback—what triggered it, what emotions surfaced, and how you felt physically. This reflection can provide insights into both your triggers and your emotional responses, equipping you with knowledge for the next time it happens. Engaging in calming activities, like listening to soothing music, can also aid in recovery; music can have a unique ability to offer a gentle escape and allow your mind to settle.

Preparation is key to managing flashbacks effectively, too. Developing a flashback response plan can provide structure and support when you need it most. You're unlikely to be able to formulate a cohesive plan when you're in the midst of a flashback itself, so take advantage of the times you're not struggling to proactively deal with the times you are. You might, for example, create a "flashback toolkit," a collection of items and strategies that bring you comfort and grounding. This might include a favorite book, a calming playlist, or a scented candle—make this personalized and based on what works for you. Having these resources readily available can make a significant difference when a flashback strikes. Sharing your plan with people you trust adds another layer of support. Let them know how they can help you, whether it's offering a listening ear or simply being present. This network can provide reassurance that you are not alone and help you deal with the aftermath of a flashback.

The nature of flashbacks is that they can feel overwhelming, but with these strategies, you can regain control and find relief. Each step you take toward understanding and managing flashbacks is a step toward reclaiming your life.

## EMOTIONAL REGULATION: BALANCING YOUR INNER WORLD

Simply put, emotional regulation is the ability to manage and respond to your emotional experiences in a healthy manner. As such, it plays a pretty significant role in maintaining mental health balance, acting as the foundation for emotional stability and resilience. When emotions are well-regulated, you can deal with life's challenges with clarity and composure, maintaining a sense of equilibrium even when things are at their toughest. Conversely, dysregulated emotions can lead you to react impulsively, heightening your stress and bringing up difficulties with relationships and decision-making.

Increasing your emotional regulation involves adopting strategies that empower you to manage your emotions effectively. Cognitive-behavioral techniques offer a practical approach to this and involve identifying and challenging the negative thought patterns that can often lead to emotional distress. If you catch yourself thinking, "I always mess up," cognitive restructuring helps you reframe this thought more positively: "I made a mistake, but I can learn from it." Emotion-focused strategies, like acceptance and mindfulness practices, can also be hugely beneficial here. Acceptance involves recognizing your emotions without judgment, allowing you to experience them fully without being overwhelmed. Mindfulness practices, meanwhile, encourage you to stay present, reducing the tendency to ruminate on past events or worry about the future.

Recognizing early signs of emotional dysregulation is the key to maintaining balance. Emotions are often accompanied by physical sensations. Here are some to watch out for:

- **A racing heart:** You might feel your heart beating faster or more irregularly. It's common to feel fluttering or pounding sensations.
- **Tightness in your chest:** There are various forms this might take, with the sensation sometimes described as pressure, squeezing, or heaviness. Note that this is different

from chest pains—which are typically a reason to immediately seek medical attention.
- **A knot in your stomach:** While this feeling differs from person to person, it typically involves an unpleasant, unsettled feeling.

By monitoring these sensations, you can identify when you're becoming dysregulated and take proactive steps to address it. Keeping an emotion diary is a valuable tool here; you use it to track mood fluctuations, noting the circumstances and triggers associated with each emotional shift. Over time, this diary becomes a resource for identifying patterns and understanding the nuances of your emotional responses—just like journaling works for figuring out triggers and dealing with flashbacks. Once you've spotted the patterns, you can anticipate and prepare for situations that might challenge your emotional regulation.

Self-care is integral to emotional regulation, too, since lifestyle choices can significantly impact your emotional health. Regular physical activity, for instance, does more than just make your body healthier; it also boost your emotional well-being. Exercise releases endorphins, the body's natural mood elevators, which help reduce stress and improve your overall mood. The exercise itself isn't limited to a specific type of physical activity; a brisk walk in the park, a yoga class, or a dance session in your living room can all be helpful. The important thing to know is incorporating any movement into your routine can make a huge difference (Mahindru, Patil, and Agrawal 2023).

Sleep and nutrition are equally important, too. Quality sleep provides your brain with the rest it needs to process emotions and maintain cognitive function, so aim for a consistent sleep schedule and create a restful environment to make your sleep quality as good as possible (Columbia Psychiatry News 2022). Nutrition, meanwhile, also plays an important role; a balanced diet rich in fruits, vegetables, and whole grains supports brain health, giving you the energy and focus needed to manage your emotions effectively (Selhub 2022).

Integrating these strategies into your life can completely alter your emotional environment, empowering you to face challenges with resilience and grace. Each step you take toward emotional regulation is a step toward a balanced and fulfilling life, where you steer your own emotions with confidence and clarity.

## THE POWER OF BREATH: BREATHING EXERCISES FOR CALM

Obviously, you need to breathe to survive. Breath, though, is more than just a biological necessity; it's a powerful tool for emotional management. Controlled breathing can heavily influence both emotional and physiological states, acting like a bridge between your mind and your body. When you control your breath, you engage your parasympathetic nervous system, which is responsible for calming the body. This system counteracts your fight-or-flight response, reducing stress and helping you calm yourself down. The science behind breath regulation highlights its calming effects, as deep, slow breaths send signals to your brain to relax and unwind. This connection between breathwork and the nervous system is hugely important, as it provides a direct method to soothe your anxiety and regain control over your emotions (Balban et al. 2023).

Various breathing exercises can offer specific benefits tailored to different emotional states and scenarios. Diaphragmatic breathing, also known as belly breathing, is particularly effective in reducing anxiety; by focusing on deep breaths that fill the diaphragm, you can lower your heart rate and promote a sense of inner calm. This technique involves placing one hand on your chest and the other on your belly, making sure that your belly rises and falls with each breath—a physical reminder of your breath's depth and power. Alternate nostril breathing, a practice rooted in yoga, balances emotions by harmonizing the left and right hemispheres of the brain. By blocking one nostril while inhaling and exhaling through the other, you create a rhythm that helps grant you equilibrium and emotional stability (Cronkleton 2024). Box breathing, often used by athletes and military personnel, boosts focus and calm by following a simple pattern: inhale for four counts, hold for four, exhale for four, and pause for four before repeating. This structured approach both calms the mind and increases concentration, making it an excellent technique for moments of stress or distraction (Stinson 2024).

Incorporating breathing exercises into your daily routine is important if you want to reap their benefits. Set aside time each day for intentional breathwork, allowing these practices to become a habitual part of your life. Using breathwork as a pre-sleep ritual can promote better rest; as you lie in bed, take long, slow breaths, focusing on the sensation of the air entering and leaving your body. This can help quiet your mind, easing your transition to sleep. Regular practice serves to both boost the effectiveness of these techniques and strengthen your ability to manage stress and emotions in the moment.

Combining breathwork with other practices can further amplify its calming effects. Pairing breathwork with guided meditations can help you with relaxation, creating a deeper state of peace and mindfulness. As you listen to a meditation, focus on your breath, allowing it to anchor you in the present moment. This combination encourages a meditative state that calms your body and mind. Similarly, using breath awareness during mindfulness exercises can help them work even better for you. As you engage in mindfulness, pay attention to the natural rhythm of your breath, noticing how it changes with your emotional state.

The power of breath is both huge and accessible, offering you a pathway to calm and balance. By integrating these exercises into your life, you cultivate a toolset that supports your emotional management and well-being. Your breath is always with you, a constant companion in your healing process—why not make use of that?

## ANGER MANAGEMENT: REFRAMING INTENSE EMOTIONS

Not all the emotions you'll have to account for when dealing with PTSD come down to the binary of depression or panic; there's also anger. It's understandable that your brain would reach for anger; it's a defense mechanism that can serve as both a shield and a sword, protecting you from perceived threats while also potentially causing harm to yourself or others. For many, anger springs from deep wells of betrayal or exploitation experienced during traumatic events. It's a physiological response that causes adrenaline to course through your veins, tensing your muscles and sending your heart racing.

These reactions are remnants of your survival instincts, designed to prepare you for fight or flight. However, in the context of PTSD, this response can become misdirected, leading to overreactions and emotional chaos that can hurt the ones you love. Anger might manifest as irritability or explosive outbursts, sometimes catching you completely off-guard. Over time, it can seep into your relationships, creating distance and misunderstanding with people you care about. Understanding the root causes of anger is really important here. For some, it might stem from past abuse or neglect, where feelings of powerlessness have festered into resentment. For others, it might be the result of ongoing stress or unmet needs. Whichever the case for you, it's important to recognize these origins to help address your anger constructively.

Managing and dealing with anger requires a varied approach, beginning with the identification of triggers and early warning signs. These might include situations, people, or even internal thoughts that spark the initial flare of anger, and by pinpointing these triggers, you can anticipate and prepare for them, reducing their impact. Physical outlets for anger, such as exercise or creative expression, are great tools; whether it's a vigorous run or a session of boxing, physical activity can channel aggression into movement, releasing built-up tension in a constructive way and restoring a sense of calm. Creative outlets like painting or writing offer a different form of release, allowing you to explore and process your emotions through art. Mindfulness exercises also play a key role, as they encourage you to sit with your anger, observe it without judgment, and understand its underlying messages. This practice can turn anger from a destructive force into a source of insight and growth.

Communication is key when it comes to expressing anger in healthy ways. Assertive communication techniques allow you to convey feelings without resorting to aggression. This involves stating your needs and emotions clearly and respectfully, using "I" statements to own your feelings rather than placing blame on other people. For example, you might use "I feel frustrated when … " instead of "You always make me angry." Active listening complements these techniques; listening with intent and empathy helps create a dialogue where all parties feel heard and valued. This approach defuses tension in the short term and strengthens relationships in the long term, turning anger into an opportunity for connection rather than conflict.

The long-term benefits of effective anger management are massive. Mastering anger can lead to significant personal growth and improved relationships. By changing how you interact with anger, you develop better self-awareness and emotional intelligence. Ultimately, these skills empower you to work through life's challenges with greater ease and resilience (even when those challenges don't directly involve anger). In essence, anger management is about reclaiming control, turning a potentially destructive emotion into a catalyst for positive change. By understanding and addressing your anger with intention and compassion, you open the door to a life where your emotions can be your allies rather than just your adversaries.

CHAPTER 4

# PRACTICAL COPING STRATEGIES FOR EVERYDAY LIFE

If you're working through the day-to-day of PTSD, one of the most important—and underrated—things you can have is a simple sense of stability. A daily routine can be a powerful anchor, offering a reliable structure that reduces anxiety and gives you back a sense of control. Establishing a consistent routine provides predictability, which isn't a bad thing, as it alleviates the uncertainty that often accompanies PTSD, helping you manage symptoms more effectively.

## THE IMPORTANCE OF A DAILY ROUTINE

Creating a daily routine begins with identifying activities that set a positive tone. Start your day with simple morning rituals that ground you; maybe this involves savoring a quiet cup of tea, spending a few moments journaling your thoughts, or engaging in gentle stretching to awaken your body. Rituals like this offer a reassuring start, and more importantly, they set the stage for a day filled with intentionality and mindfulness. Mealtimes are more important than you might think, and you'll want to set them at specific times. Scheduled meal times can serve as important touchpoints, keeping up your energy levels and providing nourishment for both your body and your mind. A nutritious breakfast, a balanced lunch, and a wholesome dinner each play a role in sustaining your well-being throughout the day, helping stabilize your blood sugar levels and reduce any mood swings.

A personalized daily schedule starts with listing your tasks and categorizing them by priority. This process helps you focus on what matters most, keeping the important activities centered with the attention they deserve. Once you've identified your priorities, don't just focus on work; incorporate breaks and leisure activities into your schedule. These moments of rest are absolutely necessary, allowing you to recharge and maintain productivity without feeling overwhelmed. Whether it's a short walk, a few minutes of meditation, or just some time to breathe, these pauses greatly boost your capacity to manage stress.

A consistent routine plays a pivotal role in reducing anxiety by offering a framework that mitigates feelings of unpredictability. It's important to remain adaptable, though, as unexpected changes are always inevitable. Develop techniques for adjusting routines when you need to, but flexibility doesn't mean abandoning your routine altogether; rather, it means being open to modifying it to accommodate life's fluctuations.

Maintaining flexibility within a structured routine is hugely important for long-term success. Strategies for balancing your routine with spontaneity can include setting aside time for unplanned activities, but the best method is just allowing for some variability within your schedule. You want your routine to be a tool for support rather than a rigid system that increases your stress levels. You'll also need to be open to changing your routine as your life changes (as with, say, a new job or a move). Don't be afraid to reassess your priorities and make adjustments as needed. Your routine should change with you, supporting your growth and resilience as you work toward healing.

*Interactive Element: Personal Routine Planner*

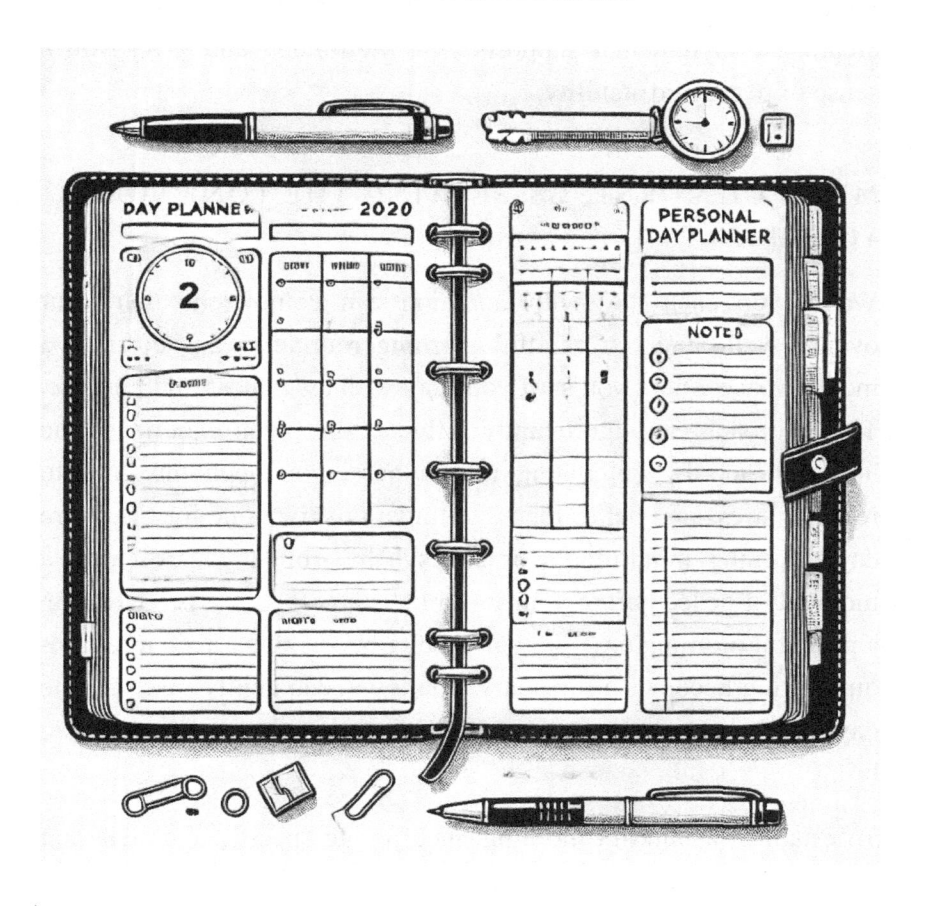

Take a moment to create your personal routine planner. List your daily activities and categorize them by priority. Identify times for meals, breaks, and leisure activities. Think about how your routine supports your goals and well-being and adjust it as needed. Use this planner as a flexible guide, adapting it to meet your changing needs and circumstances.

Incorporating these elements into your life can completely change how you deal with each day. A well-constructed routine provides a foundation for healing, empowering you to face challenges with confidence and composure. As you embrace this approach, remember that routines aren't about perfection; they're about creating a rhythm that supports your well-being and gives you a sense of peace and stability.

## MINDFUL MORNINGS: SETTING THE TONE FOR YOUR DAY

Waking up each day with intention can completely alter your overall well-being. A mindful morning routine means creating a mental space where you start your day with awareness and purpose. This approach can significantly influence how you experience the hours ahead—by cultivating mindfulness, you open the door to reduced stress and better focus, setting a positive tone for the entire day. Morning mindfulness practices help ground you, offering a moment of peace before your to-do list starts to take over. Creating a peaceful morning environment further boosts this effect, as a tranquil setting becomes a sanctuary where you can gently ease into the day, preparing your mind and body for what the day is going to bring.

To establish a mindful morning, incorporate specific activities that match your needs and preferences. A brief meditation or breathing exercise after waking up might be a good idea; this can be as simple as taking a few deep breaths while focusing on the sensations of each inhale and exhale. It's definitely a good idea to follow this with a stretching routine to awaken your body gently, especially if you're older. Stretching increases your flexibility while encouraging blood flow, energizing you for the day ahead (Stathokostas et al. 2012). Next, engage in mindful journaling to set your daily intentions. Use this time to reflect on your goals, aspirations, and emotions, and write freely, letting your thoughts flow without judgment.

The impact of mindful mornings on mental health is tremendous. Research supports how much it can help, highlighting the benefits of morning mindfulness in reducing stress and improving cognitive function. Studies show that individuals who practice mindfulness regularly experience less anxiety and greater emotional resilience, equipping them to handle the day's challenges with composure and grace (Basso et al. 2019).

Customizing your morning routine is extremely important for making sure it matters to you personally and thus effectively supports your well-being. Choose activities that engage your mind and body, such as reading a chapter from an inspiring book or sketching in a notebook; whatever you pick, the important thing is that it's something you enjoy. These activities should bring you joy and stimulate your senses, serving as a gentle nudge toward creativity and reflection. Adjust the duration and intensity of each activity based on your preferences and schedule; some mornings might call for a longer meditation session, while others might benefit from a brisk walk in the fresh air. The key is to remain flexible and attentive to your needs, allowing your routine to grow and change as you do.

A mindful morning routine is not about perfection; it's about creating a space that sets you up for a day filled with intention and purpose. By starting your day with mindfulness, you cultivate a mindset that embraces the present moment, encouraging a deeper connection to yourself and the world around you.

## WORKPLACE STRATEGIES: DEALING WITH TRIGGERS IN PROFESSIONAL SETTINGS

Experiencing a professional environment with PTSD can present unique challenges. Workplaces are filled with potential triggers that can heighten anxiety and stress levels, and compared to your personal life, you're less likely to be surrounded by people who want to support you. Deadlines can feel like looming specters, pressing down with relentless urgency, while meetings might make you feel exposed or scrutinized. Beyond these situational stressors, sensory triggers like office noise and harsh lighting can exacerbate your symptoms, making it difficult to concentrate or remain calm. Recognizing these triggers is the first step in mitigating their impact; by identifying what specifically sets off your anxiety, you can begin to strategize ways to effectively manage your stressors.

Managing workplace stress requires a whole toolkit of practical strategies. Effective time management is extremely important, as it can change how you approach tasks, reducing the chaos and anxiety of overlapping deadlines. Prioritize your workload by breaking tasks into manageable segments and setting realistic timelines for completion—it's good to push yourself, but you don't want to push yourself too hard. Creating a calming workspace can also significantly alleviate stress; personalize your desk with items that bring comfort and joy, such as a small plant or a photo of a loved one. Noise-canceling headphones can also be a great tool to block out distracting sounds, creating a bubble of peace in the midst of a bustling office.

Open communication with colleagues and supervisors is another key aspect of managing workplace triggers, as discussing your needs and boundaries can help create a supportive work environment. When disclosing PTSD in a professional setting, it's important to approach the conversation with clarity and confidence. You might say, "I sometimes experience anxiety, and certain accommodations can help me manage it effectively." Examples of supportive accommodations include flexible scheduling, the option to work from home, or access to a quiet space when needed. These adjustments can make a significant difference in your ability to manage stress and perform effectively. Remember, advocating for yourself is not a sign of weakness but a step toward creating a work environment that supports your well-being.

The nice thing about the modern age is that showing up to an office each day isn't the only option on the table. Remote work and flexible arrangements can offer additional opportunities to manage PTSD symptoms if your employer agrees to them. Setting up a home office tailored to your needs can have a huge impact on your focus and relaxation. Choose a space that minimizes distractions, and organize it in a way that promotes comfort and efficiency; this might include ergonomic furniture, soft lighting, and personal touches that make the space welcoming—the important thing, again, is that it's whatever personally appeals to you. Managing work-life balance in a remote environment, meanwhile, involves setting clear boundaries between work and personal time. Establish a routine that delineates when work begins and ends, and resist the urge to extend work hours into personal time. This separation is extremely important for maintaining mental health and preventing burnout.

Incorporating these strategies into your professional life can create a more manageable and supportive work environment. As you deal with the issues raised by PTSD in the workplace, remember that you are not alone. By recognizing triggers, employing effective management techniques, and advocating for your needs, you can create a work setting that both accommodates and empowers you.

## SOCIAL SITUATIONS: PREPARING FOR POTENTIAL CHALLENGES

Social interactions can be particularly daunting when dealing with PTSD. The thought of large gatherings can stir up a whirlwind of anxiety, as unfamiliar environments often feel overwhelming. You might have a palpable fear of being judged or misunderstood by others, and that might lead you to hesitate to even engage with social circles. You might also find yourself scanning the room for exits or rehearsing conversations in your head, worried about how you'll be perceived. This anxiety is about both the social setting itself and the potential for triggers that might fly at you out of nowhere, turning what should be a pleasant experience into a source of stress. Understanding these challenges is extremely important in preparing yourself for social situations, allowing you to engage with more confidence and less fear.

One good way to deal with these challenges is to engage in role-playing social scenarios as a practical preparation tool. Look, I know it might sound silly, but this approach can be really helpful, as it allows you to practice responses and build confidence in a safe environment. By rehearsing potential conversations or reactions, you create a mental script that can be recalled when you need it. This can reduce the uncertainty that fuels anxiety by providing you with a sense of preparedness and control.

Setting personal goals for social engagement is another effective strategy. Start small, maybe by attending a brief event or joining a small group gathering. Gradually increase your exposure as you become more comfortable, celebrating each success along the way. These goals serve as benchmarks for progress, helping you track your growth and build resilience in social settings. Social engagement is like any other muscle; the more you exercise it, the stronger it becomes.

Setting boundaries and advocating for yourself in social situations can alleviate pressure and increase your comfort, too. It's important to express your needs clearly and confidently; if an invitation feels overwhelming, it's perfectly acceptable to decline politely without guilt. You want to do so tactfully (thanking the host for the invite is always a good idea), but you also don't need to make up some excuse; "I need some time to recharge" is a completely understandable thing to say. Communicating your comfort levels with trusted friends or family can also provide support, so let them know how they can best help you, whether it's by staying close during a gathering or checking in with you afterward to see how you're doing.

After social interactions, prioritize post-social self-care to recharge and process your experiences. Quiet reflection time can be particularly beneficial, offering a chance to decompress and evaluate how you felt during the event. If you're particularly stressed by something that happened, journaling about the experience can be a good idea, as it allows you to note what went well and what you found challenging. This helps you process the event and allows you to see an overall view of what happened–both the good and the bad. Engaging in soothing activities like reading or listening to music can also help you get back into a relaxed state, letting you unwind and restoring your mental equilibrium. Choose activities that bring you peace and joy, allowing your mind to settle and rejuvenate after the social demands of the day.

Dealing with social situations with PTSD requires a thoughtful approach that balances preparation with self-compassion. By understanding your challenges, employing practical strategies, and prioritizing self-care, you can engage in social interactions with increased confidence and reduced anxiety.

## SLEEP SOLUTIONS: OVERCOMING NIGHTMARES AND INSOMNIA

Sleep is often a battleground for those living with PTSD, where the night brings not rest but a cascade of nightmares and insomnia. Trauma impacts sleep in significant ways, creating disturbances that ripple back into your daily life. You might lie awake, your mind replaying distressing memories, or drift into sleep only to be jolted awake by vivid nightmares that echo past traumas. Insomnia, the inability to fall or stay asleep, can become a relentless and extremely unwelcome companion, leaving you exhausted and on edge. These disruptions to sleep can further exacerbate PTSD symptoms, creating a feedback loop that impairs your cognitive function, mood, and overall health. You may find yourself irritable, struggling to concentrate, or feeling disconnected from the world around you. The effects of poor sleep are far-reaching, undermining your ability to cope with daily stresses and eroding your resilience over time.

Luckily, there are some tools that can help you get your sleep under control. One effective and underrated method for improving sleep quality is to establish a calming bedtime routine. This involves winding down before bed, signaling to your body that it's time to sleep. Activities that promote relaxation, such as reading a book, taking a warm bath, or practicing gentle stretches, can all be really helpful in calming your body down and transitioning your mind from the busyness of the day to a more restful state. Limiting screen time before bed is also a good idea, as the blue light emitted by screens interferes with melatonin production, the hormone responsible for regulating sleep (West et al. 2011). Set a boundary by turning off electronic devices at least an hour before bed, allowing your body to naturally prepare for sleep. Instead, turn to calming activities that don't involve screens, like listening to soothing music or practicing mindfulness meditation.

Managing nightmares, meanwhile, requires targeted approaches that address both the frequency and emotional impact of your dreams. Imagery Rehearsal Therapy (IRT) is an effective technique for re-scripting nightmares. This involves visualizing the nightmare while awake and consciously changing the ending to one that is less frightening. By practicing this altered version repeatedly, you can reduce the emotional charge associated with the nightmare, ultimately decreasing its occurrence (Stevens 2022).

Nightmares and insomnia aren't the only PTSD-related obstacles to sleep, either. Obstructive Sleep Apnea (OSA) is a condition in which someone's airway narrows or collapses at irregular intervals while they sleep. This tends to leave their sleep scattered and inconsistent, and it can even lead to serious health issues when not properly treated (Newsom and Singh 2024). For reasons unknown, OSA tends to occur more frequently in people suffering from PTSD. One of the best solutions to this problem is a continuous positive airway pressure (CPAP) machine (Pacheco and Dimitriu 2024).

Calming sleep aids like weighted blankets can also provide comfort. The gentle pressure of a weighted blanket mimics the sensation of being held, promoting a sense of safety and relaxation. This can help reduce anxiety and improve sleep quality, making it easier to fall and stay asleep. Numerous studies have actually shown that weighted blankets can improve sleep quality, even if not used for an extended period of time; one demonstrated improved sleep with as little as 30 minutes of use (Yu et al. 2024).

Creating a sleep-friendly environment can be extremely important for increasing both your comfort and general relaxation levels. There are number of ways to accomplish this:

- **Adjust the room temperature.** A cool, comfortable setting is best, since a cooler environment can promote deeper sleep (Harding et al. 2019).
- **Opt for soft, dim lights that mimic natural darkness.** This helps to regulate your body's internal clock.
- **Incorporate white noise machines or soothing sounds to further boost your sleep space.** These sounds mask disruptive noises and create a consistent auditory environment that supports relaxation. Whether it's the gentle hum of a fan or the soft patter of rain, these auditory elements can help lull you into a restful sleep.

For some people, finding a way to restful sleep can feel elusive. But by implementing these strategies, you can create an environment that nurtures rest and recovery. Each step, though simple, contributes to a greater sense of control over your sleep and well-being. As you explore these solutions, remember that patience and persistence matter; don't just try something and give up entirely. Stick with it, and eventually, you'll get there.

## NUTRITION AND PHYSICAL HEALTH: SUPPORTING YOUR MIND THROUGH BODY

The link between nutrition and mental health is just as significant as with sleep, yet it's often overlooked. What you eat can significantly impact how you feel, both emotionally and cognitively. A balanced diet supports brain function by providing important nutrients that facilitate neurotransmitter production and brain connectivity. For example, Omega-3 fatty acids, found in fish like salmon and in flaxseeds, play a surprisingly important role in mood regulation. These healthy fats increase the brain's ability to communicate effectively, reducing inflammation and potentially alleviating symptoms of depression and anxiety (Grosso et al. 2014). Omega-3s help build cell membranes in the brain and possess anti-inflammatory properties that can protect brain cells from damage (Hjalmarsdottir 2023). On the other hand, diets high in processed foods and sugars can lead to mood swings and cognitive decline by causing spikes and crashes in blood sugar levels, which can exacerbate feelings of irritability and fatigue, making it harder to cope with daily stresses (Wadyka 2024). Caffeine, too, can disrupt sleep patterns, leading to increased anxiety and mood swings (Spritzler 2023).

To support mental wellness through diet, it's important to focus on nutritious, whole foods. A variety of colorful fruits and vegetables should form the cornerstone of your meals, as they provide vitamins and antioxidants that protect your brain from oxidative stress. Leafy greens, berries, and bright orange vegetables like sweet potatoes are particularly beneficial (Jiang, Liu, and Li 2021). Whole grains and lean proteins are important, too, as they offer sustained energy, preventing the highs and lows that refined carbohydrates can cause. Nuts, seeds, and oats, along with proteins like beans and lentils, help maintain steady blood sugar levels and support neurotransmitter function, which is the key to mood regulation. Incorporating these foods into your diet can create a solid foundation for both mental and physical health (Davidson 2024). These small changes can have a big impact over time.

Additionally, try reducing your intake of processed foods, sugars, and caffeine. Swap sugary snacks for whole fruits or nuts, choose whole grains over refined ones, and go for caffeine-free drinks as much as possible. These adjustments both stabilize energy levels and promote a more balanced mood throughout the day. By paying attention to what you consume, you empower yourself to take control of your mental well-being, reinforcing your resilience against the challenges posed by PTSD.

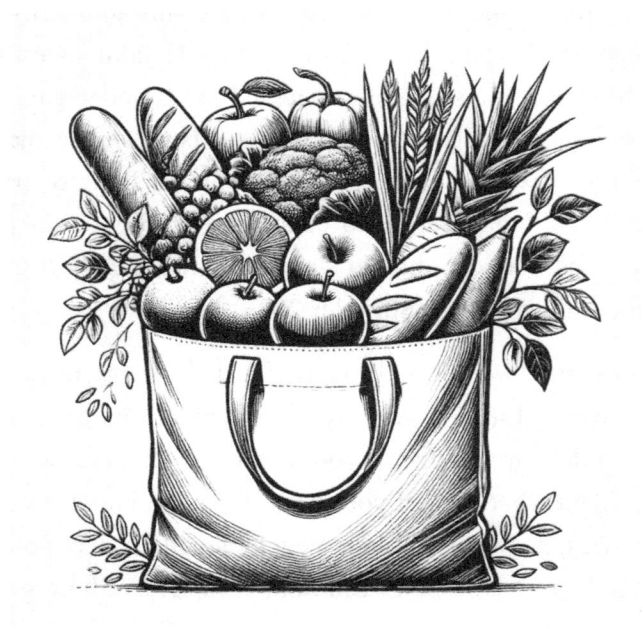

Physical activity, as we touched on briefly in Chapter 3, is another cornerstone of managing PTSD, offering a tangible way to increase your emotional stability. Exercise releases endorphins, the body's natural mood lifters, which help reduce stress and improve overall mood. Activities such as yoga and walking are particularly beneficial, as they combine physical movement with mindfulness, helping create a sense of calm and presence. Yoga, with its focus on breath and body awareness, can help release tension and promote relaxation. Walking, especially in nature, provides a change of scenery and a break from daily pressures. A lot of people find solace in activities like these, using them as coping tools to work through the emotional turbulence of PTSD.

Integrating nutrition and exercise into your daily life can feel daunting, but it starts with small, manageable steps. Meal planning is a practical approach to making sure you're engaging in balanced nutrition throughout the week. Set aside time each week to plan your meals, focusing on a variety of colorful vegetables, lean proteins, and whole grains. The added benefit here is that having meals planned out reduces the temptation to opt for less healthy choices if you don't feel like making decisions in the moment. When it comes to exercise, setting realistic fitness goals is extremely important, so start with achievable targets like a fifteen-minute walk each day or a weekly yoga class. Choosing activities you can do anytime and building up from there helps reinforce the habit, making it a natural part of your routine.

As you integrate these healthy habits, remember that nutrition and physical health are interconnected aspects of your overall well-being. By nurturing your body, you support your mind, creating a foundation for healing and resilience. These practices empower you to take proactive steps toward managing PTSD, increasing your capacity to face life's challenges with strength and clarity.

CHAPTER 5

# REBUILDING RELATIONSHIPS AND COMMUNITY

One of the worst things about PTSD is the damage it can do to the relationships around you, where the echoes of trauma can create barriers to connection. Luckily, there's often hope. The path to rebuilding relationships and community is fraught with challenges, but it is also rich with the potential for healing and growth. These relationships can serve as lifelines, offering support, understanding, and the comfort of shared experiences. However, to cultivate these connections, you first have to deal with the challenge of communication—a skill that is both an art and a necessity.

## HOW TO ESTABLISH OPEN AND CLEAR COMMUNICATION

Open and clear communication forms the cornerstone of strong relationships in general, and this is especially true if you're dealing with PTSD. Expressing your needs to loved ones requires courage and clarity. Much like when dealing with anger management, the use of "I" statements—such as "I feel overwhelmed when ... " or "I need some time to process ... "—is a powerful tool. These statements center your emotions and experiences, reducing the likelihood the person you're talking to will take them as blame and get defensive. "I" statements allow you to express your feelings without casting judgment, which helps nurture an environment of openness and respect. This shift in perspective encourages people to understand and empathize with you, which ultimately allows for healthier dialogues.

For communication to be truly effective, though, it has to be reciprocal. This means you can't only speak; you also need to actively listen—a skill that involves more than simply hearing words. Active listening requires presence and attention in order to make sure you fully comprehend what the other person is trying to convey. Reflective listening exercises can boost this skill; try summarizing what you've heard and then confirming it with the speaker, as in, "So you're saying that you feel anxious when ... ?" This has the added benefit of validating the speaker's feelings, reinforcing their importance and value in the conversation. Techniques like these build trust, as they demonstrate a genuine effort to connect and empathize with the other person's perspective.

I remember when my partner and I struggled with communication over how to deal with our childrens' various conflicting activity schedules. Figuring out who would take which kid where and when felt like trying to solve a math problem–and neither of us are exactly "numbers" people. Through a commitment to "I" statements and active listening, though, we were ultimately able to find a way to resolve our issues and strengthen our relationship in the process.

Our secret was ultimately empathy. Empathy is the core of pretty much all meaningful communication. Empathy involves acknowledging and accepting your own emotions, as well as creating a safe space for others to do the same. Recognizing and validating your loved ones' feelings is a key component of empathy. When you say, "I understand why you feel this way," and offer support rather than solutions or judgments, it allows people to feel like you're really hearing them. This acknowledgment can be incredibly healing, as it assures the other person that their emotions are valid and respected.

Dealing with difficult conversations is often inevitable, but with the right strategies, they, too, can be approached with grace and understanding. Setting ground rules for respectful communication is a proactive step; agreeing to listen without interrupting, to speak without raising voices, and to avoid accusatory language can create a foundation for a constructive conversation. If emotions become overwhelming in the heat of the moment, taking breaks can provide necessary respite, allowing both parties to regroup before continuing the conversation. This pause is not an avoidance; it's a strategic tool to maintain integrity and respect between the two of you. Approaching these conversations with the intention of understanding, rather than winning, helps create a collaborative atmosphere where you seek solutions together rather than try to impose them unilaterally.

In the context of rebuilding relationships and community, you need to remember that communication is about creating connections, understanding, and empathy. Through thoughtful communication, relationships can become sources of healing and support, offering the strength and resilience needed to deal with the challenges of living with PTSD.

## TRUST AND INTIMACY: RE-ESTABLISHING CONNECTIONS

The thing about trust is it's difficult to build and easy to lose. Once compromised, trust can be challenging to rebuild, especially after trauma has driven a wedge between you and those you hold dear. The path to restoration—as much as it's possible—begins with acknowledging past breaches of trust and understanding their impact. It's important to recognize how these breaches have shaped current relationship dynamics. Acknowledging what happened is less about dwelling on the past than it is about creating a shared understanding of where you've been. This mutual recognition lays a foundation for setting realistic expectations, knowing that rebuilding trust is a gradual process, one that requires patience from all parties involved. Rather than an overnight fix, rebuilding trust is a commitment to consistent and honest communication, where each small step forward is a victory worth celebrating.

Intimacy, both emotional and physical, thrives on a foundation of trust. To strengthen these connections, it can help to engage in shared activities that promote bonding. Maybe this involves taking a walk together, cooking a meal, or just sharing a quiet moment over a cup of tea; the important thing isn't the activity itself but what it can do for your relationships. These moments of togetherness can help rebuild connections, providing opportunities for forming closer bonds. Vulnerability is hugely important here—showing you trust someone with your honest, authentic self works wonders to encourage people to trust you in return. This openness may seem daunting, but it can ultimately deepen the intimacy of your relationships and form the core of trust-building.

Barriers to trust and intimacy are often rooted in fear—fear of rejection, fear of being misunderstood, fear of reliving past trauma.

These fears are valid, but letting them rule you ultimately only impedes the growth of relationships if they're left unaddressed. It's important to recognize how past traumas can act as barriers, making closeness feel risky or even impossible. Understanding these fears and addressing them openly with trusted loved ones can begin to break down these walls. Your goal is to create a space where fears can be expressed without judgment and where they can be examined and understood. This isn't about eliminating fear because you can't just shut fear down and pretend it isn't there. Instead, your goal is to learn to work through your fears together, using the process as a stepping stone toward greater connection and healing.

My own trauma led me to repeatedly reject and push away those who only wanted to help. My brother in particular wanted so badly to help me overcome my PTSD, but time and time again, I lashed out at him. I felt unworthy of love and support, and I wound up damaging our once-close relationship in the process. Fortunately, I eventually got the help I needed, and I was able to rebuild our relationship slowly over time.

That's the most important thing to remember: none of this is going to happen in a day. Rebuilding connections isn't a solitary endeavor but a collaborative effort, requiring commitment and understanding from everyone involved. Allow yourself to lean on those who offer you support, and be open to the moments of vulnerability and courage that come up along the way. While the process may be challenging, it's also a testament to the strength and resilience inherent in the human spirit.

## GENDER-SPECIFIC CHALLENGES IN RELATIONSHIPS

It's a bit of an understatement to say that instilled gender roles can impact the way people express emotions and connect with others. Societal expectations have long imposed a narrow framework on emotional expression, particularly for men, who are often encouraged to suppress their emotions as vulnerability becomes equated with weakness. This pressure can stifle emotional intimacy, creating a barrier in relationships where open communication is especially important. On the other hand, women may face societal expectations that demand emotional availability and nurturing—sometimes at the expense of their own needs. These deeply ingrained roles can lead to misunderstandings and unmet expectations within relationships.

While emotionally stifling concepts of how different genders are supposed to behave might make things difficult, there's still hope. These challenges are not insurmountable; they just require awareness, dialogue, and a commitment to change to work through effectively. Understanding these gender-specific issues is extremely important if you want to form a more equitable relationship where both partners feel valued and understood.

Gender massively shapes the experience of trauma and recovery from PTSD. For many men, the expectation to remain stoic can lead to internalized stress and a reluctance to seek help. This suppression of emotions doesn't help; you can't push down your feelings forever. Instead, it can ultimately exacerbate PTSD symptoms as unresolved feelings linger beneath the surface, intensifying your anxiety and isolation. Vulnerability is the culprit here; men are frequently taught that vulnerability means weakness and thus might find it challenging to express. The fear of judgment or rejection makes sense within society's imposed framework, but it can also hinder the healing process.

Conversely, women often face unique vulnerabilities in intimate relationships, which are frequently the root of the trauma itself. Experiences of abuse or violation can deeply and understandably affect trust and intimacy, making it difficult to feel safe and secure with a partner. In addition, women are significantly more likely to deal with PTSD during their lives; roughly 10 percent of women experience PTSD compared to 4 percent of men (Vernor 2019). Recognizing these gender-specific impacts, though, allows for a tailored approach to healing, one that respects and acknowledges the distinct experiences of every gender and nurtures a supportive environment for recovery.

If you want to resolve these issues, you're going to have to talk about them; working through gender-specific challenges requires open discussions about gender roles and expectations within relationships. Encouraging these conversations can also illuminate assumptions and biases that may be influencing behavior and interactions. It's important to create a safe space where both partners can express their feelings and concerns without fear of criticism or dismissal. In some cases, seeking gender-sensitive therapy or support groups can help a lot, as these resources offer a platform for people to explore their experiences in a supportive environment, surrounded by others who can relate to their challenges. Therapy can also provide valuable insights and strategies for overcoming gender-related hurdles, promoting a sense of empowerment and confidence in dealing with your issues.

Overcoming gender-specific challenges in relationships is not without its obstacles, but by embracing open dialogue, seeking support, and promoting inclusivity, you can create a path toward deeper connection and understanding. These efforts require patience and persistence, but the reward of a relationship where both partners feel heard, understood, and valued ultimately speaks for itself. Dealing with the concept of gender in relationships means you have to remain committed to creating an environment of empathy and respect where everyone involved can thrive.

## BUILDING YOUR SUPPORT NETWORK: FINDING YOUR TRIBE

In the midst of healing from trauma, the power of a supportive network can often be the determining factor in how smooth the process goes. Friends, family, and community are frequently our anchors in turbulent times, providing both emotional comfort and practical assistance in helping with tasks when the weight of the world feels too heavy. A close friend might offer a listening ear during moments of distress, while a family member might assist with daily chores, giving you the space to breathe and heal. These acts of kindness, though seemingly small, can have a tremendous impact on your process toward wellness.

Identifying potential members of your support network requires a keen understanding of trustworthiness and reliability because you need to know who you can count on. It's important to assess relationships honestly, thinking about who has consistently shown up for you in times of need. Look for those who have proven themselves to be empathetic and understanding—they're the ones most likely to offer you genuine support. Initiating connections with potential allies can be daunting, but it's an important step, as a simple message or phone call expressing a desire to reconnect or seek support can open doors to deeper connections. Be honest about your needs and intentions, allowing others to step into roles they are comfortable with. Remember, a support network is not about quantity but quality; even a few reliable friends can make a significant difference. Conversely, a hundred friends don't mean anything if none of them will show up when you need them.

A diverse support system offers a wealth of benefits, including emotional, informational, and practical support. It's valuable to have friends who can offer a variety of perspectives and strengths, from those who can provide emotional comfort to others who might share helpful resources or advice. Balancing close friendships with broader community involvement, such as joining local clubs or groups, can also enrich your personal network. This diversity means you're not reliant on a single source for support, reducing the pressure on any one individual and creating a more sustainable emotional ecosystem.

Active participation in your support network is important for it to succeed. Regularly attending local events or support groups can reinforce connections and provide continuous encouragement. These gatherings offer opportunities to share experiences, learn from others, and deepen relationships. Involvement doesn't only mean receiving support; offering help and encouragement to others is just as important. Whether it's offering a ride, lending an ear, or simply checking in, these gestures contribute to a supportive and nurturing community—remember that you'll get back what you give. Engaging actively keeps your network resilient, ready to offer support in times of need.

Building a support network is more than just collecting people like stamps or playing cards; it involves creating genuine connections based on trust, empathy, and mutual respect. By thoughtfully choosing allies and engaging actively, you create a community that supports both your healing and your growth. This network becomes an integral part of your life, offering strength and companionship as you work through the difficulties of recovery. Through this collective support, you find resilience and hope, knowing that you are not alone in healing.

## THE ROLE OF ONLINE COMMUNITIES IN HEALING

We live in a world where the concept of community has now expanded far beyond physical borders, offering new avenues for connection and support. Online support communities have emerged as absolutely necessary lifelines for many people, providing a platform where individuals can share their experiences, seek advice, and find solace in the company of others who understand their struggles in a way people never could before the rise of the internet. These virtual spaces offer the benefits of anonymity and accessibility, allowing you to connect with others without the fear of judgment or the constraints of geography. Being able to talk to anyone at any time from the comfort of your own home ultimately makes support available whenever you need it most. Popular online forums and social media groups, such as Reddit's r/PTSD or Facebook support groups, have become havens for those seeking understanding and companionship in their healing process.

But dealing with these virtual environments comes with its own set of challenges. The anonymity that provides you comfort can also potentially open the door to misinformation and negative interactions. Not everyone online has good intentions, and the risk of encountering harmful advice or toxic behavior is real. To protect yourself, it's important to approach these communities with caution. Establish clear boundaries to maintain your mental well-being, and be mindful of how much time you spend online to avoid burnout. It's easy to become overwhelmed by the constant influx of information and stories, so take breaks when needed and engage in activities that replenish your energy. You also have to watch out for misinformation; not only is it prevalent online, but "verified" users (the ones often regarded as the most trustworthy) are frequently the worst culprits for spreading untruths (Temple Now 2021).

Finding the right online community can be as personal as finding a therapist. Before joining, research the community's guidelines and values to make sure they match your needs and expectations. Look for spaces that prioritize respect and empathy, where members are encouraged to share their experiences and offer support in a constructive manner. Once you've found a community that feels right, think about how you can actively contribute because sharing your own experiences can be empowering and may help others feel less alone. Offering support to others strengthens the community and often feels deeply rewarding; don't underestimate how helping people feels good in and of itself.

## HEALING WITH EMPATHY: HELPING OTHERS UNDERSTAND WHAT YOU'RE GOING THROUGH

There are a lot of ways to describe empathy, but ultimately, the important thing is it allows us to see the world through another person's eyes. This ability to understand and share the feelings of others is paramount in relationships, especially when you're dealing with the aftermath of PTSD. Empathy serves as a bridge that connects seemingly disparate experiences, allowing people to connect with experiences they themselves have not felt. It plays an important role in reducing conflict, as understanding the emotional undercurrents of a disagreement can change a confrontation into a cooperative problem-solving session. When you approach situations with empathy, discussions shift from adversarial to collaborative, creating a space where both parties feel valued and heard. This mutual respect lays the groundwork for more supportive relationships, where the focus is on understanding and meeting each other's needs.

Educating others about PTSD is an important step in nurturing empathy. When those around you understand the intricacies of PTSD, they are better equipped to offer support and compassion. Creating informational materials or presentations can be an effective way to communicate your experiences, since these resources can provide an overview of what PTSD entails, its symptoms, and its effects on your daily life. Sharing educational resources about PTSD can also offer insight into what PTSD means and dispel some common myths that surround it. By providing loved ones with the knowledge they need, you empower them to help you with your own healing.

Empathy is reciprocal by nature; you have to extend it to others in order to be able to seek it in return. This means actively listening to and validating the experiences of those around us, acknowledging their emotions and perspectives. Encouraging open dialogue and mutual learning enriches relationships, allowing for a more nuanced understanding of each other's worlds. This exchange of empathy creates a cycle of support, where both parties feel seen and valued. Healing thus becomes a collective endeavor where empathy acts as the balm that soothes and strengthens the bonds between us.

As you work empathy into our relationships, you lay the groundwork for a more compassionate and connected world. This process is not without its challenges, but the potential rewards are absolutely massive. By nurturing a process for empathy, we open the door to deepening our relationships, creating a network of emotional connections that uplifts and empowers us.

CHAPTER 6

# HARNESSING THE POWER OF NARRATIVE AND STORYTELLING

Sometimes, it's not enough to be able to tell people you're suffering; you have to tell them in a way that, emotionally, they simply can't ignore. This is where the power of narrative and storytelling comes into play. Accounts of struggle and survival have the power to captivate people in a way dry facts often don't, and the act of storytelling is ultimately a powerful offering of vulnerability and strength. Sharing your personal narrative can be an immensely beneficial tool for healing, helping you externalize internal experiences by taking the fragmented pieces of trauma and shaping them into a coherent and meaningful story. This process can help reduce feelings of shame and correct unhelpful beliefs about the event, giving you a sense of mastery over your own experiences. By articulating your story, you take control of the narrative.

An important point about storytelling as a tool is that it can apply to many different types of mental health issues. This isn't a bad thing, as other mental health issues are often comorbid issues with PTSD

(Brady et al 2000). Instead, view these techniques as a therapeutic option for various things you might be struggling with.

## SHARING YOUR STORY

If done well, the act of sharing your story is going to build empathy and understanding among your listeners. When you open up about your experiences with true vulnerability and openness, you invite others into your world. This shared understanding can help create a sense of solidarity as listeners recognize parts of themselves in your story. They connect with the emotions and challenges you've faced, creating a bridge of empathy that transcends individual differences. This connection can be deeply healing for both the storyteller and their listeners. By giving voice to your experiences, you contribute to a collective narrative of resilience and compassion, demonstrating that no one is alone in their struggles.

Vulnerability is the cornerstone of storytelling, and it requires a courageous leap into the unknown. Sharing your story exposes your inner world to the scrutiny of others—a prospect that can be tremendously daunting but which also holds the potential for empowerment. By overcoming your fear of judgment, you can find strength in your authenticity, embracing your unique experiences as part of your identity. This courage can, in turn, inspire others, encouraging them to share their own narratives and nurturing a culture of openness and acceptance. Creating safe environments for sharing narratives is the key part of this process, as spaces like these offer a refuge where individuals can speak freely, knowing they will be met with understanding and compassion rather than judgment and derision. Whether it's a support group, a close-knit circle of friends, or a therapist's office, safe environments provide the security needed to explore and express personal truths.

Finding your voice and expressing your unique narrative can be an arduous task in and of itself. Journaling exercises that encourage self-reflection can help, so try writing about your experiences, emotions, and the lessons you've learned along the way. This practice allows you to explore the nuances of your story, identifying key themes and messages that wind through your experience. As you write, pay attention to the patterns that emerge—moments of triumph and struggle that define your narrative. Identifying these elements can help you build a story that is both authentic and impactful.

***Journaling Prompt: Uncovering Your Story***

Take a moment to reflect on a pivotal experience in your life. Write about the emotions, challenges, and insights that emerged from its aftermath. Think about how the experience has shaped you and what message you wish to convey through your story. Use this prompt as a starting point to uncover the layers of your narrative, embracing both the light and shadow that have defined what you've been through. *Please note that a Journaling Prompt page has been included in the downloadable work book at the end of the book.*

***Reflection Section: Your Resilience Toolkit***

Take a moment to reflect on your experiences with adversity and think about the strategies you've used to deal with these challenges. Write down three techniques that have helped you build resilience. Then, reflect on the role of community in your life; how have shared experiences and support from others influenced your healing process? Use this reflection to create a personal resilience toolkit, incorporating the strategies and support networks that empower you personally. *A Reflection Section page has been included in the downloadable work book at the end of the book.*

## STORYTELLING WORKSHOPS: CREATING YOUR NARRATIVE

Storytelling workshops offer a unique opportunity for you to develop and refine your personal narrative, turning raw experiences into compelling stories. The structure itself is designed to encourage growth and understanding. They typically begin with a warm welcome—setting a tone of safety and openness—and then participants are encouraged to share their stories in a supportive environment, where feedback is an integral part of the process. The objectives extend beyond mere storytelling; your goal is to workshop a compelling narrative while building confidence, boosting your communication skills, and deepening your understanding of your own experiences.

The collaborative nature of storytelling workshops provides an environment where stories can really breathe. Within these spaces, you're not alone; you are part of a litany of voices, each contributing to a rich, collective narrative. This collaboration allows for a diversity of perspectives, offering insights that might not surface if you were by yourself. The benefits are manifold: you gain the courage to voice your story while learning from the narratives of others, and everyone else gains the same. This shared experience nurtures both empathy and solidarity in a space where you can witness the power of your words and the impact they have on others, reinforcing the value of your experiences and the importance of sharing them with others.

If you're interested in participating or organizing a workshop, there are some steps you can take to get started. Research local or online options like libraries, community centers, and online platforms that frequently host events like these. If you're inclined to organize one, it's important to focus on creating a nurturing space. Think about the physical setting itself—comfortable seating, warm lighting, and a quiet atmosphere can really deepen and strengthen the experience. Set clear guidelines that emphasize respect, confidentiality, and constructive feedback. Participants should listen actively and engage with empathy; each story needs to be met with understanding and support. Facilitating a space where stories can be shared without fear of judgment is the key to achieving the full potential of these workshops.

## CREATING A NARRATIVE WORTH TELLING

Creating a compelling narrative, meanwhile, involves honing specific storytelling skills. Storyboarding is a good place to start as an invaluable tool for organizing and structuring your narrative. Visualize the arc of your story, identifying key moments and transitions; this process helps you focus on the elements that drive your narrative forward and which keep up a coherent and engaging flow. Sensory details can further boost your storytelling; paint vivid pictures with words, describing what happened while digging deep into how things felt, looked, and sounded. The more intricate details you can bring in, the more it will draw listeners into your story, allowing them to experience it alongside you. By engaging the senses, you breathe life into your narrative, making it connect on a deeper level with your listeners.

Feedback and revision are hugely important for refining your story. Embrace the iterative nature of storytelling and understand that every draft is a step toward clarity and impact—you're not going to get things perfect on the first try, and that's ok. In workshops, in particular, constructive feedback can serve as a mirror, reflecting back the strengths and areas for growth in your narrative. When you're giving feedback, focus on specific elements and offer constructive suggestions for making things better. When receiving feedback, listen with an open mind and really think about how the suggestions match your intentions for the story. This process polishes your narrative while honing your ability to communicate effectively, teaching you to view your story from multiple angles and enriching its depth and meaning.

**Interactive Element: Storyboarding Exercise**

Take a moment to sketch out a storyboard for your narrative. Figure out the key moments and emotions you want to convey, then think about how these elements connect to each other and flow into a larger story. Use this storyboard as a guide to shape and refine your story, making sure it captures the essence of your experiences and the message you wish to share.

## WRITING AS THERAPY: UNLEASHING YOUR INNER AUTHOR

Writing offers a unique path to self-discovery and emotional processing. The act of putting pen to paper (or fingers to keyboard) allows you to explore and understand complex emotions in a way that spoken words often can't illuminate. Writing provides a safe space to confront thoughts and feelings without fear of judgment. As you write, you may find that emotions you didn't even know you had suddenly come to the surface, offering you a look into your inner world you never even realized you needed. This process can be surprisingly cathartic, serving as a release valve for pent-up emotions. The act of writing ultimately helps to externalize your internal experiences, making them more tangible—and thus, more manageable. By seeing your thoughts laid out in front of you, you gain a new perspective, which can be the first step in healing.

Structured writing exercises can enable you to really reach the therapeutic potential of writing. Free writing is a powerful tool to unleash subconscious thoughts. Set a timer for a few minutes and write continuously without worrying about grammar or coherence; let your thoughts flow freely, capturing whatever comes to mind. Often, this exercise reveals patterns and themes that might be hidden beneath the surface, providing clarity and understanding you wouldn't have achieved just from thinking about things consciously. There are, however, more active approaches to figuring these things out, as reflective writing is another technique that aids in processing past experiences. The goal here is to dig into specific memories, examining how they have shaped your present. Through reflection, you can begin to reframe these experiences, turning them from sources of pain into chapters of growth.

Establishing a personal writing practice requires commitment and intention. Start by setting goals for your writing sessions; decide how often you want to write and what you hope to achieve by doing so. Whether it's daily journaling or weekly reflective essays, having a clear purpose can motivate you to keep going. Creating an inspiring and comfortable writing environment, meanwhile, removes another hurdle from the process. Maybe this is a cozy corner in your home or a quiet spot in a park. Whatever you choose, be sure to surround yourself with elements that nurture your creativity, like soft lighting or calming music. This dedicated space becomes a sanctuary where you can explore your thoughts without distraction.

Don't dismiss the importance of what you have to share with the world; your words hold value, and your story deserves to be shared. Explore opportunities to publish your personal stories, whether through blogs, online platforms, or traditional publishing routes. Sharing your writing with others both amplifies your voice and connects you with a wider audience who may find solace and inspiration in your experiences. Celebrate the completion of writing projects, too—no matter how small—as each finished piece is a testament to your resilience and growth. These milestones are worthy of acknowledgment, marking your progress and the courage it took to express your truth. Don't be afraid to encourage yourself for what you've already achieved.

The path from writing for personal reflection to becoming an author involves embracing your narrative as a meaningful contribution. Your story, with all its nuances and complexities, can serve the purpose of hope and understanding for other people who connect with it. By sharing your writing, you're contributing to your healing —but you're also offering a lifeline to others dealing with similar challenges.

## CHANGING TRAUMA INTO TRIUMPH

Narrative plays an important role in reframing trauma, offering a lens through which individuals can reinterpret their experiences. Many find strength in techniques like re-authoring personal narratives, shifting the focus from victimhood to agency. By identifying growth opportunities within traumatic experiences, individuals can uncover aspects of resilience they may have overlooked.

Reflecting on personal achievements can reveal the resilience and fortitude that trauma often obscures. Human minds have a natural tendency to focus on negative emotions in what's known as "Negativity Bias." Steps need to be taken to avoid falling into that trap. Journaling prompts can serve as a guide in this process. Write about moments where you overcame challenges, noting how you managed to deal with your struggles. Celebrate milestones in your healing process, no matter how small, as each step forward is a testament to your strength and determination. By acknowledging these victories, you reinforce a narrative of resilience and growth, shifting focus from what was lost to what you've gained. This practice bolsters your own self-esteem and inspires others to see the potential for triumph in their own lives (Cherry 2023).

Personal stories also hold the potential to spark broader social change, connecting individual narratives to collective movements. Many advocacy and awareness initiatives are born from the courage of individuals who share their experiences. Survivors who speak out against violence or discrimination, using their stories to challenge societal norms and inspire reform, can have a tremendous impact. These narratives serve to both empower the storyteller and galvanize communities to action, nurturing a sense of empathy and understanding. As readers, sharing your story can contribute to this ripple effect. By adding your voice to the chorus, you participate in a larger dialogue that promotes healing and change. Your story, with its unique perspective, can illuminate paths of possibility for others, reinforcing the notion that personal growth can lead to societal progress.

CHAPTER 7

# LONG-TERM WELLNESS AND RESILIENCE

So, let's talk about resilience. Resilience in humans is essentially an ability to withstand and grow from life's challenges. It doesn't mean simply bouncing back–instead, resilience is the capacity to emerge stronger, wiser, and more compassionate. Resilience plays an important role in recovery from trauma, enabling you to deal with adversity with fortitude and flexibility, turning obstacles into stepping stones for growth. By cultivating resilience, you can face life's uncertainties with a steady heart and an open mind, finding balance in the midst of chaos (Snijders et al. 2018).

## RESILIENCE IN EVERYDAY LIFE

Resilience, for me, has always been about refusing to give up, no matter how tough things got. I had to get my first job when I was just 10 years old, after my parents divorced. I worked to buy clothes and pay for extra-curricular activities. As I grew older, I juggled school and multiple jobs. It wasn't easy, but I held onto the belief that if I could just keep moving forward, I could overcome the obstacles in my path and create a better future for myself. Resilience wasn't about avoiding struggles—it was about facing them head-on and finding the strength to rise above.

That mindset gave me hope, even during the hardest times. It helped me stay optimistic, cope with stress, and bounce back from setbacks. Resilience became my foundation, the thing that kept me grounded and gave me the confidence to tackle life's challenges. It taught me how to find emotional balance in the chaos and focus on my goals, no matter how far away they seemed. By committing to resilience, I turned my struggles into stepping stones, knowing that every small step forward was bringing me closer to the success I was determined to achieve.

Building resilience involves practical strategies that increase your capacity to adapt and thrive, and cultivating a growth mindset is the first part of the process. This mindset, rooted in the belief that abilities and intelligence can be developed, encourages positive self-talk and a focus on learning from experiences. By viewing challenges as opportunities for growth, you shift from a fixed mindset—where obstacles are insurmountable—to one that embraces change and progress. Engaging in challenging activities also creates resilience; problem-solving tasks, creative pursuits, or physical challenges push you beyond your comfort zone, building confidence and resilience over time. These activities teach perseverance and adaptability, reinforcing your ability to tackle life's hurdles.

Adversity is often painful, but it can also be a powerful catalyst for resilience. Facing challenges head-on increases your ability to deal with them head-on in the future, fueling personal growth and turning your hardships into sources of strength. Think about an athlete who, after a career-ending injury, channels their passion into coaching and inspires others, or the entrepreneur who, after a failed business venture, learns lessons that lead to future success. Adversity can totally alter your worldview by refining and strengthening your character. Reflecting on past experiences allows you to gain valuable insights that bolster your resilience, equipping you to deal with future challenges.

Ongoing practice and reflection are an important part of reinforcing resilient behaviors, too. Journaling is a powerful tool for tracking resilience development because writing about challenges and triumphs helps you gain clarity and perspective. Journaling prompts such as "What did I learn from this experience?" or "How did I adapt to change?" encourage introspection and growth. These reflections will also help you spot patterns, revealing areas where resilience has been successfully applied or where you might want to work to strengthen it. Creating a "resilience toolkit" further supports this practice; fill it with reminders of past successes, inspirational quotes, or strategies that have helped you persevere. This toolkit serves as a tangible resource, reinforcing your resilience and reminding you of your capacity to overcome adversity.

## *Reflection Section: Cultivating Resilience*

Take a moment to reflect on a recent challenge you faced. Write down the lessons you learned and how you adapted; what strategies did you use to overcome obstacles, and how did those strategies contribute to your resilience? Add these reflections to your "resilience toolkit" as a reminder of your strength and growth.

As you continue on this path, remember that resilience is not a destination but a muscle you build up over time, cultivated through practice, reflection, and a commitment to growth. By embracing resilience, you empower yourself to work through life's complexities with grace and strength, finding beauty and meaning in the midst of adversity.

## PREPARING FOR POTENTIAL RELAPSES: STRATEGIES FOR STABILITY

The path to recovery is often lined with unexpected challenges, and setbacks are a natural—albeit frustrating—part of the healing process. It's important to grasp that relapses do not erase progress; instead, they are opportunities to learn and strengthen your resilience. Slipping up once doesn't mean you've permanently ruined all the hard work you've done. Moreover, relapses are not failures; they are a reminder that healing is a process with ebbs and flows. By normalizing relapses as a part of recovery, you can alleviate the shame and guilt that often accompany them. This gets right back to the idea of self-compassion we talked about in Chapter 2; if you'd grant grace to someone else who is struggling, why wouldn't you grant it to yourself?

It's also important to understand what might have caused the relapse in the first place. Common triggers for setbacks might include stress, fatigue, or encountering reminders of past trauma. Even significant life changes, whether positive or negative, can destabilize the progress you've made. Recognizing these triggers and understanding their potential impact is the first step in mitigating their effects—and in not blaming yourself too harshly for relapsing in the first place.

To effectively manage relapses, a proactive approach is absolutely necessary, and developing a relapse prevention plan tailored to your unique experiences can minimize the impact of setbacks. This plan should include specific coping strategies to address triggers head-on. Identify the warning signs that often precede a relapse; these might be emotional signals, like increased irritability or anxiety, or physical symptoms, such as disrupted sleep patterns or headaches. By pinpointing these signs early on, you can implement strategies to prevent a full-blown relapse. Engaging in relaxation techniques, reaching out to a trusted friend, or revisiting therapeutic practices can ultimately help you regain—and keep—control. Building a support network is equally important because everyone needs a safety net during moments of vulnerability. Surround yourself with individuals who understand your healing process and can provide encouragement and guidance when you need it.

Regular self-assessment is another great way to strengthen your relapse prevention. Incorporating routine self-check-ins into your schedule allows you to monitor your mental health and make necessary adjustments. These assessments can be as simple as asking yourself how you're feeling each day, what challenges you might face, and how you plan to address them; it might take some tinkering to figure out what works best for you, so don't be afraid to experiment. Early intervention is key when warning signs appear, but luckily, you've got options to deal with them based on whatever works for you. Whether it's practicing mindfulness, engaging in physical activity, or seeking professional help, taking action can prevent a temporary setback from escalating. This proactive stance empowers you to take charge of your recovery, reinforcing your commitment to well-being.

Amidst this focus on prevention, you can never forget the importance of self-compassion. It's easy to be hard on yourself when faced with setbacks, but treating yourself with kindness is absolutely necessary for the healing process. Always remind yourself that being human means encountering obstacles and that each challenge is also an opportunity for growth. Affirmations and mantras can reinforce this mindset, offering comfort and encouragement.

Phrases like "I am doing my best, and that's enough" or "Every step, no matter how small, is progress" can shift your internal dialogue toward positivity and self-acceptance.

### Reflection Section: Dealing with Setbacks

Pick up your journal again and reflect on a time when you faced a setback in your recovery. What triggers or signs did you notice beforehand? How did you respond to the situation? Write down the strategies that helped you regain your footing and think about how you can incorporate them into your relapse prevention plan moving forward.

Meanwhile, think about starting a lifestyle journal. Each day, note one positive action you've taken toward your well-being. It could be a healthy meal, a mindful moment, or a restful night's sleep. Reflect on how these actions make you feel and their impact on your overall wellness. Over time, this journal will become a great resource for you to look back on your progress and encourage yourself.

Incorporating lifestyle changes requires patience and self-compassion. It's important to remember that progress is often gradual, and setbacks are part of the process. Embrace each step forward as a victory, and approach challenges with a sense of curiosity and openness.

## CREATING A BALANCE: INTEGRATING WORK, LIFE, AND HEALING

It's important not to simply tip over in one direction or another when it comes to your personal life; if you want to really achieve the best results in dealing with your PTSD, you'll need to balance your work, your personal life, and the activities you undertake specifically for the purposes of healing. Achieving equilibrium among these areas is absolutely necessary for reducing stress and promoting mental health. When things are out of balance, the consequences can ripple across your life, manifesting as chronic stress, burnout, and emotional exhaustion—not exactly a list of things you want to use to describe yourself. These imbalances can erode your mental health, while what you want is to find the sort of harmony that nourishes every part of your life.

My sister is a nurse, and she takes it seriously as a caregiver who gives tirelessly to others. I admire her tremendously for it, but her fatal flaw is that she often neglects to replenish her own well-being. More than once, she's come close to complete burnout until myself or our brother stepped in to convince her to take a break and recharge her batteries. I worry frequently about her capacity to keep going when she struggles to find the right balance between the various aspects of her life.

Setting boundaries is a fundamental strategy for achieving work-life balance. Boundaries signify where your professional life ends and your personal life begins, encouraging you to disconnect from work emails after hours or to carve out time each day solely for self-care. Prioritizing self-care activities within your daily routine is equally important. It doesn't matter whether it's a daily walk, a meditation session, or simply sitting quietly with a cup of tea—these moments of care are not indulgences but necessities for maintaining balance. They replenish your mental and emotional reserves, equipping you to engage more fully with both work and personal life.

Work environments play a significant role in shaping mental health, with supportive settings contributing greatly to your healing. Workplaces that promote well-being often implement policies designed to reduce stress and encourage a healthy work-life balance—maybe they offer flexible work hours, provide mental health days, or encourage open dialogues about mental health concerns. These policies create a culture of support, allowing employees to feel valued and understood. If you work from home, creating a supportive home office environment can really increase your well-being. Designate a specific area for work that separates professional responsibilities from personal spaces. Make sure this area is well-lit and comfortable, and incorporate elements that promote calm, like soothing artwork or greenery (plants can have healing properties, like we talked about in Chapter 2). This separation helps maintain focus during work hours while allowing you to truly relax once the workday ends.

Reflection and adjustment of priorities are ongoing processes in maintaining balance. Assessing your current balance involves taking a step back to evaluate how your time and energy are currently being distributed. Are work commitments overshadowing personal relationships? Is self-care being sidelined in favor of professional responsibilities? Reflection exercises can help clarify these questions, guiding you to realign priorities in a way that supports your overall well-being.

Strategies for delegating tasks and managing responsibilities, meanwhile, can ease the burden of imbalance. At work, this might mean sharing duties with colleagues or learning to say no when your plate is full. At home, it could involve enlisting family members to share household tasks or seeking external help when needed. By delegating, you alleviate a lot of the pressure you might be feeling, allowing yourself the space to focus on what truly matters.

Balance is a constantly changing state, ever-shifting with the demands of daily life. Embrace this evolution as a fluid process that adapts to your changing needs and circumstances. Think about what brings you joy and what fulfills you, and make sure these elements become a key part of your routine. This holistic approach to balance recognizes the interconnectedness of work, life, and healing, each element feeding into and supporting the others. As you cultivate this balance, you create a foundation that both sustains your mental health and enriches your entire life experience.

## EMPOWERMENT THROUGH SELF-ADVOCACY: CLAIMING YOUR RIGHTS

Self-advocacy is the act of taking control of your life by clearly expressing your needs, desires, and rights. It's about being your own champion and speaking up for what you need to thrive. In many contexts, such as healthcare or the workplace, self-advocacy involves communicating with professionals who can influence your well-being. For instance, in a medical setting, self-advocacy might mean asking your doctor questions to fully understand your treatment options. In the workplace, it could involve discussing necessary accommodations with your supervisor to ensure you can perform your best. The psychological benefits of self-advocacy are substantial. By taking charge, you affirm your self-worth, build confidence, and cultivate a sense of empowerment. It's an exercise in self-respect, teaching you that your voice matters and that you deserve to be heard.

Effective self-advocacy requires preparation and strategy. Before entering a meeting or discussion, clarify your goals and the points you wish to convey. It might be a good idea to write them down so you have a clear roadmap to guide the conversation. Practicing assertive communication techniques is also important. These techniques involve expressing your thoughts and needs confidently and respectfully without aggression or passivity, so use "I" statements to articulate your perspective, as in, "I need more flexibility in my work schedule to manage my health." Understanding your legal rights, particularly related to mental health and accommodations, further strengthens your position, so familiarize yourself with relevant laws and policies. The Americans with Disabilities Act (ADA) mandates reasonable workplace accommodations for individuals with mental health conditions and is a great resource to call on to get a recalcitrant workplace to grant you the accommodations you're owed (Parker 2022). This knowledge equips you with the tools to advocate effectively and make sure your needs are met.

Despite its benefits, self-advocacy is not without challenges. Fear of judgment or backlash can deter you from speaking up, especially if past attempts to do so were met with resistance or misunderstanding. These fears are common, but you can still address them through practice and positive reinforcement. Start advocating for yourself in low-stakes situations, gradually building your confidence; with each successful interaction, your self-assurance will grow, reinforcing your ability to advocate in more complex scenarios. Self-advocacy is a skill, and like any skill, it improves with practice. Positive experiences where your needs are acknowledged and respected will bolster your confidence, encouraging you to advocate for yourself even more in the future.

Building a support network can significantly boost your self-advocacy endeavors. Seek out individuals or organizations that share your goals and values; people in a similar situation can offer guidance, share resources, and provide moral support. Local advocacy groups or online communities focused on mental health can be invaluable sources of encouragement and information. They can offer insights from their own experiences, helping you refine your strategies and approach. This exchange of knowledge and support creates a collaborative environment where everyone benefits.

Self-advocacy is a powerful tool for personal empowerment. It allows you to take control of your life and make sure your needs and rights are recognized and respected. Through preparation, practice, and support, you can confidently communicate your needs, paving the way for a life that aligns with your values and aspirations. Embrace self-advocacy as an ongoing process that changes with your experiences and growth. As you advocate for yourself, you achieve the dual aims of empowering your own healing and inspiring others to find their voice and claim their rights.

## CELEBRATING PROGRESS: ACKNOWLEDGING YOUR ACHIEVEMENTS

Recognizing personal achievements may seem like a navel-gazing act of self-congratulation, but that's not the case at all. Instead, it's a necessary component of long-term healing and growth. Celebrating progress reinforces your motivation to keep going and boosts your self-esteem, providing tangible evidence of your capabilities and resilience. When you acknowledge your accomplishments, no matter how small, you cultivate a positive self-image, fueling continued growth and instilling a sense of pride in how far you've come. There's a huge psychological uplift that accompanies the successful completion of even minor tasks, like sticking to a new routine or successfully dealing with a challenging social situation. These moments, though they may seem trivial, are milestones worth celebrating, each a stepping stone toward greater accomplishments.

Tracking progress can be an empowering practice, offering a clear view of the strides you've made. One creative way to achieve this is by maintaining a "success journal" where you regularly document your achievements and reflect on what you've learned along the way. This journal becomes a personal testament to your growth, a record you can use to revisit your accomplishments and draw inspiration from them. Planning small celebrations to reach specific goals is another good idea. These celebrations don't need to be grand; a simple treat or a day spent doing something you love can serve as a meaningful acknowledgment of your hard work. Marking these moments reinforces the value of your efforts and the importance of recognizing success along the way.

Don't be afraid to take the time to reflect on what you've already achieved, even as you're in the midst of healing. Reflection exercises can help you evaluate personal change, prompting questions like, "What have I learned from this experience?" or "How have I changed since I began?" Additionally, sharing stories of change with supportive individuals can make this reflection do even more for you. By articulating what you've been through to others, you both celebrate your progress and strengthen your connections with those who support you. Their feedback and encouragement can provide new perspectives on your achievements, further validating your efforts and reinforcing your growth.

Gratitude plays a significant role in celebrating success, shifting your focus from what remains to be done to what you've already achieved. Keeping a gratitude journal centered on personal achievements encourages this mindset. Each entry might highlight accomplishments and the factors that contributed to them, nurturing a sense of appreciation for how far you've come and the support you've received along the way. Expressing gratitude to those who have been part of your process is equally important. Whether it's a heartfelt note or a simple thank you, acknowledging how others have contributed to your healing reinforces the bonds that have supported your progress thus far. Gratitude enriches the celebration of success, making it a shared experience that honors both individual and collective achievements.

Celebrating progress is an ongoing practice involving a conscious decision to pause and recognize the value of your efforts. Celebrating like this increases your self-awareness and encourages your continued growth, reminding you that progress is not always linear —but it *is* always happening. As you celebrate your achievements, you affirm your resilience and commitment to change, keeping the ball rolling on future success.

CHAPTER 8

# LOOK TOWARD A HOLISTIC APPROACH TO HEALING

PTSD isn't just about what happens in your brain; your mind and body are inextricably connected, both from trauma and in the process of healing from that trauma. For me, PTSD is triggered by the smell of fire, and the sirens that come with it. That moment of sensory overload triggers my heart racing, shoulders tensing, andmy breath shortening; this is the mind-body connection in action —a powerful interplay where mental and physical states influence each other. This connection highlights the significance of a holistic approach to healing, one that recognizes the symbiotic relationship between your thoughts, emotions, and physical sensations. Stress, for example, often manifests physically through muscle tension, headaches, and digestive issues. These symptoms are your body's way of communicating that something is wrong, urging you to pay attention to both the mental and physical cues it's trying to send you.

## HOW YOUR EMOTIONS IMPACT YOUR HEALTH

Emotional well-being also plays a pivotal role in physical health, impacting indicators like blood pressure and immune function (Schaare et al. 2023; D'Acquisto 2017). When you're emotionally balanced, your body's ability to maintain homeostasis is significantly greater. Conversely, prolonged emotional distress can lead to higher blood pressure, reduced immune response, and increased vulnerability to illness. Recognizing this relationship invites a more comprehensive approach to managing PTSD, where addressing emotional health concurrently supports physical recovery. You can't ignore either aspect of healing; you have to consider both at once.

The concept of the mind-body connection is not new. Many cultures have long recognized its importance, integrating it into their healing practices. Traditional Chinese Medicine (TCM), with a history spanning over 2,000 years, exemplifies this holistic perspective, linking specific emotions to corresponding organs and suggesting that imbalances in one can affect the other. Anger, for instance, has long been associated with the liver, while fear is related to the kidneys. This understanding informs TCM's approach, which includes acupuncture and herbal remedies to restore this balance (Pacific College 2014). Similarly, indigenous Native American medical practices sometimes emphasize harmony between mind and body, often using rituals and natural remedies to align the spirit with physical wellness (Koithan and Farrell 2010). Healing encompasses more than just the absence of symptoms–of equal importance is achieving equilibrium.

To empower the mind-body connection, various techniques can be incorporated into your daily routine. Mindfulness-Based Stress Reduction (MBSR) practices are particularly effective in promoting awareness of the present moment and reducing stress responses (this also makes MBSR a great help for dealing with chronic illnesses). Through mindfulness meditation, you learn to observe your thoughts and bodily sensations without judgment, nurturing a sense of calm and clarity (Niazi and Niazi 2011). Progressive muscle relaxation is another valuable tool, guiding you to systematically tense and release muscle groups, linking physical relaxation with mental ease. This practice alleviates tension while heightening body awareness, helping you recognize and address stress signals early (Nunez 2020).

Adopting a holistic approach to healing offers numerous benefits—both emotional and physical. It increases self-awareness, allowing you to identify patterns and triggers that contribute to stress, which in turn empowers you to make informed choices, whether that means adjusting your environment or seeking social support. Holistic practices also improve emotional regulation, helping you respond to challenges with greater composure. On a physical level, these practices support cardiovascular health, improve immune function, and boost your overall vitality. By integrating mind and body practices in your healing, you cultivate a balanced state that supports sustained recovery and well-being.

*Reflection Section: Exploring Your Mind-Body Connection*

Take a moment to reflect on how stress affects your body. Do you notice tension in your shoulders or an unsettled stomach during anxious moments? Write down these observations and think about how they relate to your emotional state. Next, choose a mindfulness or relaxation technique to practice this week. Document your experiences and any changes you notice in your physical and emotional responses when engaging in them. This exercise encourages a deeper understanding of your mind-body connection, guiding you toward a more holistic approach to healing.

## INTEGRATING YOGA AND MOVEMENT: A PATH TO SERENITY

When you face the start of a new day, you're going to want your body to be full of anticipation and readiness to embrace the world. For many of us that may seem impossible, but it's actually well within our grasp. This sense of tranquility can come from the practice of yoga and movement, which offer tremendous benefits for mental health. Yoga, for instance, is a powerful tool in reducing anxiety and elevating mood, dissipating tension, and instilling a sense of calm through its combination of physical postures, breath control, and meditation. When you engage in yoga, you allow your body to release pent-up stress, creating space for peace and clarity (Nyer et al. 2018).

Yoga isn't the only option for physical activity that boosts mental health; rhythmic movements, such as Tai Chi or walking, can also serve as meditative practices in motion. These activities both soothe the mind and increase emotional well-being by promoting the release of endorphins, the body's natural mood elevators. The gentle, flowing movements of Tai Chi, in particular, encourage balance and introspection, nurturing a serene state of mind that can be carried throughout your day (Sani et al. 2023).

The beauty of yoga and movement healing practices lies in their diversity, allowing you to choose styles that match your personal needs and preferences. Vinyasa flow, known for its energetic transitions, offers a vigorous workout that invigorates the body and mind. It is ideal for those who seek to channel their energy into a structured practice, finding empowerment in each pose (Pizer 2024). On the other hand, restorative yoga focuses on deep relaxation and stress relief. With its emphasis on long-held poses and breathing, restorative yoga nurtures the nervous system, inviting a sense of calm and rejuvenation (Lindberg 2020). For those desiring a more expressive outlet, dance movement therapy provides a creative way to explore emotions through movement. This therapy encourages self-expression and helps release emotional blockages, offering a liberating experience that can be both healing and joyful (Lindberg 2023).

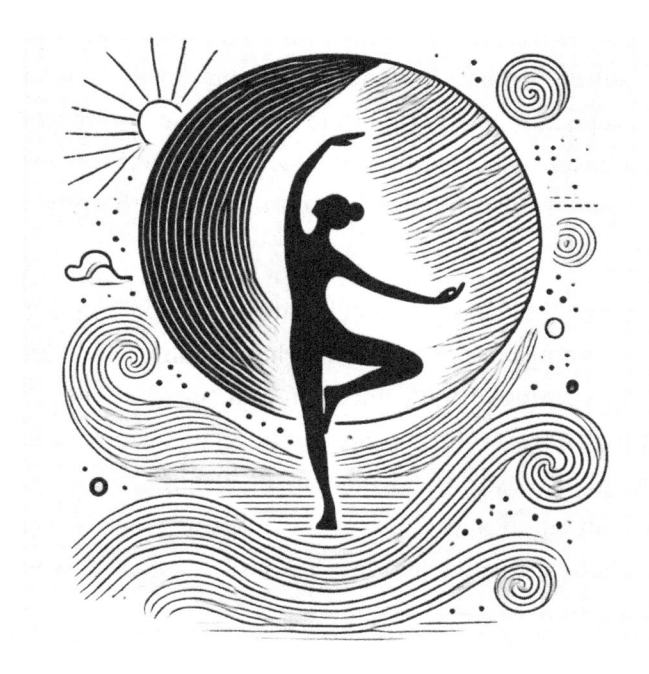

Incorporating these practices into daily life requires both intention and forethought. Setting up a home yoga practice can be a practical approach, particularly with the abundance of online resources available. Platforms offering guided sessions make it easier than ever to practice yoga in the comfort of your own space—on your schedule. It's a good idea to create a weekly movement schedule that balances different activities to keep your routine engaging and varied. You might dedicate certain days to yoga while reserving others for walks in nature or Tai Chi sessions. This variety serves to both prevent monotony and keep you engaging with different muscle groups and mental states.

Breath plays an important role in increasing the benefits of movement practices, acting as the bridge between your body and your mind. In yoga, deep, intentional breathing increases your focus, grounding you in the present moment and intensifying your practice's effectiveness. As you inhale, feel the expansion of your chest and the resulting infusion of energy; as you exhale, release tension and invite relaxation. This rhythmic breathing can turn your movement practice into a meditative experience where each breath and movement align harmoniously, nurturing both physical and emotional health.

Through these practices, you cultivate a deeper connection with yourself, nurturing an environment where healing and serenity can flourish. As you move with intention and breathe with awareness, you open pathways to greater emotional resilience and inner peace. This integration of yoga and movement becomes more of a sanctuary for your mind and body, a place where you can find refuge from the challenges of everyday life and embrace the tranquility that resides within.

## MEDITATION PRACTICES: FINDING PEACE WITHIN

Meditation invites you to step into a space of stillness, where the noise of the outside world fades and inner calm takes precedence. The goals of this practice are inner peace and emotional stability, offering a refuge that reduces your stress and increases your relaxation. Regular meditation increases your focus, allowing your thoughts to become clearer, like a still pond reflecting a tranquil sky. Through meditation, you cultivate a state of tranquility that can ripple throughout your life, bringing clarity and balance to your daily experiences.

There are various meditation techniques, and each offers a unique path to inner peace. Mindfulness meditation focuses on present-moment awareness, encouraging you to observe your thoughts and sensations without judgment. This practice helps you detach from the whirlwind of daily stresses, grounding you in the here and now (Cherry 2024). Loving-kindness meditation, on the other hand, nurtures your compassion by guiding you to send wishes of well-being to yourself and others, changing feelings of isolation into connection and empathy (Hofmann, Grossman, and Hinton 2011). Guided imagery, meanwhile, relies on visualization, using detailed mental images to promote relaxation and healing (West 2022). These techniques offer diverse avenues for exploration, allowing you to choose practices that match your personal goals and preferences.

To begin a meditation practice, start by setting up a dedicated meditation space at home. This space serves as a physical reminder of your commitment to mindfulness, offering a refuge from everyday distractions. Much like your home office, decorate it with items that inspire peace, such as candles, cushions, or calming artwork. Starting with short, guided sessions can help build confidence, providing structure and support as you acclimate to the practice. As you grow more comfortable, gradually increase the duration of your practice, allowing yourself to dive deeper into the meditative experience.

Ultimately, consistency is the cornerstone of making sure you get the most out of meditation. Creating a meditation schedule that fits your lifestyle helps encourage regular practice, reinforcing the habit and deepening its impact. The time of day is less important than its consistency; whether you choose to meditate in the morning to set a peaceful tone for the day or in the evening to unwind, the idea is to integrate meditation into your daily routine. It might also be a good idea to keep a meditation journal to track your progress and experiences. Documenting your sessions allows you to reflect on changes in your mental state, helping you understand how meditation influences your emotional well-being. This practice of self-reflection also increases your self-awareness, helping you recognize patterns and growth over time.

## MINDFUL EATING: FEEDING YOUR BRAIN

Mindful eating completely changes your relationship with food, encouraging you to savor each bite and recognize your body's cues. It involves being present during meals, appreciating the flavors and textures of your food, and acknowledging the nourishment it provides. This practice can help prevent overeating and promote a balanced diet. It's a good idea to start with practicing gratitude before meals, a simple act of acknowledging the effort that went into bringing food to your table. As you eat, focus on the sensory experience—the colors, aromas, tastes, etc. This presence allows you to tune into hunger and fullness signals, guiding you to eat when you're hungry and stop when you're satisfied. Over time, mindful eating helps create a healthier relationship with food, reducing stress around meals and increasing your overall enjoyment.

Certain foods, meanwhile, are particularly beneficial for brain health and mood enhancement. We covered some of these back in Chapter 4, but let's go over a few more now. Blueberries are rich in antioxidants that support cognitive function. These tiny fruits help combat oxidative stress and inflammation, both of which can affect brain health. A handful of blueberries in your morning cereal or smoothie can be a delicious way to give yourself a brain boost (Khalid et al. 2017). Dark chocolate, often seen as an indulgence, also has mood-boosting properties due to its ability to increase endorphin production. A small piece of dark chocolate can provide a comforting boost, lifting your spirits while satisfying your sweet tooth (Nehlig 2013).

Think about your current eating habits and how they might influence your mood and energy. Are there small changes you can make to incorporate more brain-boosting foods into your diet? Each choice, though small, contributes to the larger picture of your mental health.

## ENGAGING IN CREATIVE THERAPIES: ART AND MUSIC

Creative expression offers another pathway to emotional healing, allowing you to explore and process feelings that words alone can't capture. Art therapy, for instance, provides a safe space to convey complex emotions through visual mediums, and studies have shown art therapy can be tremendously effective in treating mental health (Shukla et al. 2022).. Whether it's through painting, drawing, or sculpting, art becomes a conduit for translating internal experiences into tangible forms. This process facilitates emotional release while helping you discover subconscious patterns that might be influencing your well-being (Psychology Today Staff 2022). Similarly, music therapy harnesses the power of sound to reduce your anxiety and boost your mood. Engaging with music—it doesn't matter if it's by listening, playing an instrument, or composing—can evoke memories and emotions, helping you process them in a supportive environment (Jacobson 2024).

Various forms of artistic expression offer therapeutic benefits, each providing a unique pathway to emotional release. Painting and drawing serve as powerful tools for channeling emotions, allowing you to explore feelings in a visual and tactile manner. The act of creating with your hands can also be meditative, helping nurture a sense of calm and focus. Music and dance, on the other hand, engage the body in a form of embodied storytelling. Music offers solace and connection through rhythm and melody, while dance allows you to express emotions physically, moving through space to tell your story without uttering a single word. Both mediums engage the senses, creating an immersive experience that can help process trauma.

To incorporate art into your healing, think about creating an art journal to document your emotional environment. This personal space serves as a visual diary where you can freely sketch, paint, or collage your thoughts and feelings. An art journal allows you to explore themes and patterns, offering insights into your emotional state over time. Participating in community art projects can also nurture connection and support, offering opportunities to engage with others who share similar experiences to your own. These projects often involve collaborative efforts, where each participant contributes to a larger piece of art. This shared endeavor builds community while providing a sense of belonging as you work alongside others to create something meaningful.

Collaborative art projects hold immense potential for healing, bringing individuals together in a spirit of unity and creativity. Group art workshops, for example, provide a space for participants to explore their creativity while engaging with others. These workshops often involve guided activities that encourage reflection and expression, encouraging a sense of camaraderie among participants. As you create alongside others, you may find that the shared experience offers comfort and validation, reinforcing the idea that you are not alone in your struggles. Through collective creative expression, you build connections through the universal language of art. Whether contributing to a community mural or participating in a group sculpture, these collaborative efforts remind you of the strength found in togetherness and the healing power of art.

## CREATIVE ARTISTIC THERAPY OPTIONS

Various creative therapy modalities exist to cater to different interests and needs. Painting workshops, for example, focus on self-expression, encouraging participants to explore their feelings through color and form. These sessions often emphasize process over product, allowing you to experiment without the pressure of creating a masterpiece. Group music therapy sessions offer a communal space where individuals can connect through shared musical experiences. These gatherings help nurture a sense of community and support as participants find solace in the collective harmony of sound.

Accessing creative therapies is more accessible than you might think, as many local and online programs offer workshops and sessions tailored to various artistic disciplines. Researching options in your area or exploring virtual platforms can connect you with opportunities to engage in creative expression. If you can't get to formal sessions, think about setting up a personal creative space at home. This could be a corner of a room dedicated to your artistic pursuits, complete with art supplies, musical instruments, or whatever else you need. Creating this space allows you to engage in creative activities at your own pace, helping encourage consistent practice that can be both therapeutic and enriching.

Creativity plays a huge role in personal growth, helping to nurture resilience and self-discovery. Engaging in creative activities encourages experimentation and playfulness, helping you break free from rigid thought patterns and embrace new perspectives. As you explore different mediums, you may uncover hidden talents and insights, gaining a deeper understanding of your emotional ecosystem. Reflecting on what you've learned through creative endeavors can often lead to incredible realizations, as the process of creation often mirrors that of healing. These activities also nourish the soul, providing a sense of accomplishment and fulfillment that extends beyond the creative realm.

## CONCLUSION

At the heart of what I've been trying to tell you is a vision—one that can empower you to walk the terrain of PTSD with compassion and strength. The goal has never been to "fix" what is not broken but to integrate all parts of your being, recognizing the strength and wisdom that come from your lived experiences.

Now, as you stand at this crossroads, I urge you to take the next step in your healing process. It might be a good idea to join a support group where you can share your experiences and learn from others. Start a daily mindfulness practice to anchor yourself in the present moment. Maybe you'll even want to share your story, whether through writing or conversation, to inspire and connect with others who may be on a similar path.

Community plays an important role in healing. Whether through online platforms, local groups, or community events, connecting with others who understand what you're dealing with can offer invaluable support. Shared experiences help create a sense of belonging, reminding you that you are not alone. Together, you can build a network of resilience and hope.

Looking forward, I encourage you to hold onto hope for the future. Healing from PTSD is about growth as much as it is about overcoming difficulties. Picture a future where resilience and peace are within your reach, bolstered by the tools and knowledge you've gained from this book. Remember, resilience is not about being unbreakable as much as it is about developing the strength to bend and adapt, emerging stronger and wiser.

Before we part, I want to express my deepest gratitude for your courage and commitment to healing. It takes immense bravery to confront trauma and seek growth. Know that you are supported as you keep working to heal from PTSD, and I invite you to continue engaging with resources and communities that click with you. Whether that involves following my work or joining a dedicated online community, know that support is always within your reach.

Remember that healing is a journey, not a destination. It requires patience, self-compassion, and the willingness to embrace all facets of who you are. As you move forward, carry with you the lessons you've learned; may they serve as guiding lights, illuminating your path to resilience and peace.

SCAN HERE FOR YOUR BONUS
PTSD WORK BOOK

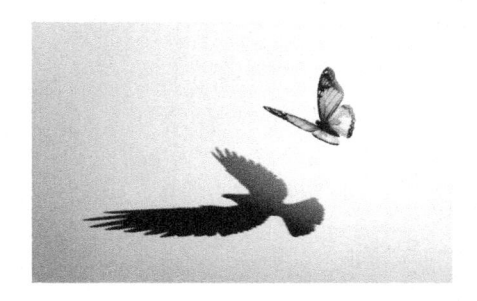

# REFERENCES

"What Is EMDR Therapy and Why Is It Used to Treat PTSD?," *American Psychological Association*, December 21, 2023. Accessed on December 18, 2024. https://www.apa.org/topics/psychotherapy/emdr-therapy-ptsd.

Anand, Kuljeet Singh and Vikas Dhikav. 2012. "Hippocampus in Health and Disease: An Overview." *Annals of Indian Academy of Neurology* 15(4): 239–46. Accessed on December 18, 2024. https://doi.org/10.4103/0972-2327.104323.

Balban, Melis Yilmaz, Eric Neri, Manuela M. Kogon, Lara Weed, Bita Nouriani, Booil Jo, Gary Holl, Jamie M. Zeitzer, David Spiegel, and Andrew D. Huberman. 2023. "Brief Structured Respiration Practices Enhance Mood and Reduce Physiological Arousal." *Cell Reports Medicine* 4(1): 100895. Accessed on December 20, 2024. https://doi.org/10.1016/j.xcrm.2022.100895.

Basso, Julia C., Alexandra McHale, Victoria Ende, Douglas J. Oberlin, and Wendy A. Suzuki. 2019. "Brief, Daily Meditation Enhances Attention, Memory, Mood, and Emotional Regulation in Non-Experienced Meditators." *Behavioural Brain Research* 356 (1): 208–20. https://doi.org/10.1016/j.bbr.2018.08.023.

Cherry, Kendra. "What Is the Negativity Bias?," *Verywell Mind*, November 13, 2023. Accessed on December 25, 2024. https://www.verywellmind.com/negative-bias-4589618.

Cherry, Kendra. "What to Know About Mindfulness Meditation," *Verywell Mind*, May 14, 2024. Accessed on December 27, 2024. https://www.verywellmind.com/mindfulness-meditation-88369.

"Amygdala," *Cleveland Clinic*, Last reviewed on April 11, 2023. Accessed on December 18, 2024. https://my.clevelandclinic.org/health/body/24894-amygdala.

Columbia Psychiatry News. "How Sleep Deprivation Impacts Mental Health," *Columbia University Department of Psychiatry*, March 16, 2022. Accessed on December 20, 2024. https://www.columbiapsychiatry.org/news/how-sleep-deprivation-affects-your-mental-health.

Corliss, Julie. "What is Cognitive Behavioral Therapy?," *Harvard Health Publishing*, June 5, 2024. Accessed on December 18, 2024. https://www.health.harvard.edu/blog/what-is-cognitive-behavioral-therapy-202406053047.

Cronkleton, Emily. "10 Breathing Exercises to Try When You're Feeling Stressed," *Healthline*, May 17, 2024. Accessed on December 20, 2024. https://www.healthline.com/health/breathing-exercise.

D'Acquisto, Fulvio. 2017. "Affective Immunology: Where Emotions and the

Immune Response Converge." *Dialogues in Clinical Neuroscience* 19(1): 9–19. Accessed on December 27, 2024. https://doi.org/10.31887/DCNS.2017.19.1/fdacquisto.

Davidson, Katey. "9 Healthy Foods That Lift Your Mood," *Healthline*, November 14, 2024. Accessed on December 27, 2024. https://www.healthline.com/nutrition/mood-food.

Grosso, Giuseppe, Fabio Galvano, Stefano Marventano, Michele Malaguarnera, Claudio Bucolo, Filippo Drago, and Filippo Caraci. 2014. "Omega-3 Fatty Acids and Depression: Scientific Evidence and Biological Mechanisms." *Oxidative Medicine and Cellular Longevity* 2014: 313570. Accessed on December 21, 2024. https://doi.org/10.1155/2014/313570.

Harding, Edward C., Nicholas P. Franks, and William Wisden. 2019. "The Temperature Dependence of Sleep." *Frontiers in Neuroscience* 13: 336. Accessed on December 21, 2024. https://doi.org/10.3389/fnins.2019.00336.

Harrison, Stephanie. "What Does Self-Compassion Really Mean?," *Harvard Business Review*, December 12, 2022. Accessed on December 18, 2024. https://hbr.org/2022/12/what-does-self-compassion-really-mean.

Haupt, Angela. "Your Houseplants Have Some Powerful Health Benefits," *Time*, March 2, 2023. Accessed on December 18, 2024. https://time.com/6258638/indoor-plants-health-benefits/.

Hjalmarsdottir, Freydis. "17 Science-Based Benefits of Omega-3 Fatty Acids," *Healthline*, January 17, 2023. Accessed on December 27, 2024. https://www.healthline.com/nutrition/17-health-benefits-of-omega-3.

Hofmann, Stefan G., Paul Grossman, and Devon E. Hinton. 2011. "Loving-Kindness and Compassion Meditation: Potential for Psychological Interventions." *Clinical Psychology Review* 31(7): 1126–1132. Accessed on December 27, 2024. https://doi.org/10.1016/j.cpr.2011.07.003.

Jacobson, Christina. "How CSU Educators are Changing Lives Through Music Therapy," *CSU Magazine*, January 17, 2024. Accessed on December 27, 2024. https://engagement.source.colostate.edu/music-therapy/.

Jiang, Shuai, Hui Liu, and Chunbao Li. 2021. "Dietary Regulation of Oxidative Stress in Chronic Metabolic Diseases." *Foods* 10(8): 1854. Accessed on December 27, 2024. https://doi.org/10.3390/foods10081854.

Khalid, Sundus, Katie L. Barfoot, Gabrielle May, Daniel J. Lamport, Shirley A. Reynolds, and Claire M. Williams. 2017. "Effects of Acute Blueberry Flavonoids on Mood in Children and Young Adults." *Nutrients* 9(2): 158. Accessed on December 27, 2024. https://doi.org/10.3390/nu9020158.

Koithan, Mary and Cynthia Farrell. 2010. "Indigenous Native American Healing Traditions." *The Journal for Nurse Practitioners* 6(6): 477–478. Accessed on December 27, 2024. https://doi.org/10.1016/j.nurpra.2010.03.016.

Lindberg, Sara. "The Benefits of Restorative Yoga and Poses to Try," *Healthline*, September 23, 2020. Accessed on December 27, 2024. https://www.healthline.com/health/restorative-yoga-poses.

Lindberg, Sara. "What Is Dance Therapy?," *Verywell Mind*, November 22, 2023. Accessed on December 27, 2024. https://www.verywellmind.com/dance-therapy-and-eating-disorder-treatment-5094952.

Maercker, Andreas, Marylene Cloitre, Rahel Bachem, Yolanda R. Schlumpf, Brigitte Khoury, Caitlin Hitchcock, and Martin Bohus. 2022. "Complex Post-Traumatic Stress Disorder." *Lancet* 400(10345): 60-72. Accessed on December 18, 2024. https://doi.org/10.1016/S0140-6736(22)00821-2.

Mahindru, Aditya, Pradeep Patil, and Varun Agrawal. 2023. "Role of Physical Activity on Mental Health and Well-Being: A Review." *Cureus* 15(1): e33475. Accessed on December 20, 2024. https://doi.org/10.7759/cureus.33475.

McFarlane, Alexander C. 2010. "The Long-term Costs of Traumatic Stress: Intertwined Physical and Psychological Consequences." *World Psychiatry* 9(1): 3-10. Accessed on December 18, 2024. https://doi.org/10.1002/j.2051-5545.2010.tb00254.x.

Murphy-Oikonen, Jodie, Karen McQueen, Ainsley Miller, Lori Chambers, Alexa Hiebert. 2020. "Unfounded Sexual Assault: Women's Experiences of Not Being Believed by the Police." *Journal of Interpersonal Violence* 37(11-12): NP8916-NP8940. Accessed on December 18, 2024. https://doi.org/10.1177/0886260520978190.

"Post-Traumatic Stress Disorder," *National Institute of Mental Health*, Last Reviewed January, 2025. Accessed on December 18, 2024. https://www.nimh.nih.gov/health/topics/post-traumatic-stress-disorder-ptsd.

Nehlig, Astrid. 2013. "The Neuroprotective Effects of Cocoa Flavanol and Its Influence on Cognitive Performance." *British Journal of Clinical Pharmacology* 75(3): 716–727. Accessed on December 27, 2024. https://doi.org/10.1111/j.1365-2125.2012.04378.x.

Newsome, Rob and Abhinav Singh. "Obstructive Sleep Apnea," *Sleep Foundation*, April 16, 2024. Accessed on January 7, 2025. https://www.sleepfoundation.org/sleep-apnea/obstructive-sleep-apnea.

Niazi, Asfandyar Khan and Shaharyar Khan Niazi. 2011. "Mindfulness-Based Stress Reduction: a Non-Pharmacological Approach for Chronic Illnesses." *North American Journal of Medicine and Science* 3(1): 20–23. Accessed on December 27, 2024. https://doi.org/10.4297/najms.2011.320.

Nunez, Kirsten. "The Benefits of Progressive Muscle Relaxation and How to Do It," *Healthline*, August 10, 2020. Accessed on December 27, 2024. https://www.healthline.com/health/progressive-muscle-relaxation.

Nyer, Maren, Maya Nauphal, Regina Roberg, and Chris Streeter. 2018. "Applications of Yoga in Psychiatry: What We Know" *Focus* 16(1): 12-18. Accessed on December 27, 2024. https://doi.org/10.1176/appi.focus.20170055.

Orbanek, Stephen. "Study Shows Verified Users Are Among Biggest Culprits When it Comes to Sharing Fake News," *Temple Now*, November 9, 2021. Accessed on December 24, 2024. https://news.temple.edu/news/2021-11-09/study-shows-verified-users-are-among-biggest-culprits-when-it-comes-sharing-fake.

Pacheco, Danielle and Alex Dimitriu. "PTSD and Sleep," *Sleep Foundation*, Last updated January 3, 2024. Accessed on January 7, 2024. https://www.sleepfoundation.org/mental-health/ptsd-and-sleep

Pacific College. "Emotions and Traditional Chinese Medicine," *Pacific College of Health and Science*, September 5, 2014. Accessed on December 27, 2024. https://www.pacificcollege.edu/news/blog/2014/09/05/emotions-and-traditional-chinese-medicine.

Parker, Kathleen D. "An Invisible Epidemic: Navigating Mental Health Issues in the Employment Relationship," *American Health Law*, August 1, 2022. Accessed on December 27, 2024. https://www.americanhealthlaw.org/content-library/connections-magazine/article/56437975-7efc-4500-976c-d2ca3ca82a39/an-invisible-epidemic-navigating-mental-health-iss.

Pizer, Ann. "Introduction to Vinyasa Yoga," *Verywell Fit*, June 10, 2024. Accessed on December 27, 2024. https://www.verywellfit.com/introduction-to-vinyasa-flow-yoga-4143120.

Psychology Today Staff. "Art Therapy," *Psychology Today*, Last reviewed on August 29, 2022. Accessed on December 27, 2024. https://www.psychologytoday.com/us/therapy-types/art-therapy.

Raypole, Crystal. "30 Grounding Techniques to Quiet Distressing Thoughts," *Healthline*, January 29, 2024. https://www.healthline.com/health/grounding-techniques.

Sani, Norliyana Abdullah, Siti Suhaila Mohd Yusoff, Mohd Noor Norhayati, and Aida Maziha Zainudin. 2023. "Tai Chi Exercise for Mental and Physical Well-Being in Patients with Depressive Symptoms: A Systematic Review and Meta-Analysis." *International Journal of Environmental Research and Public Health* 20(4): 2828. Accessed on December 27, 2024. https://doi.org/10.3390/ijerph20042828.

Schaare, H. Lina, Maria Blöchl, Deniz Kumral, Marie Uhlig, Lorenz Lemcke, Sofie L. Valk, Arno Villringer. 2023. "Associations Between Mental Health, Blood Pressure and the Development of Hypertension." *Nature Communications* 14: 1953. Accessed on December 27, 2024. https://doi.org/10.1038/s41467-023-37579-6.

Selhub, Eva. "Nutritional Psychiatry: Your Brain on Food," *Harvard Health Publish-*

*ing,* September 18, 2022. Accessed on December 20, 2024. https://www.health.harvard.edu/blog/nutritional-psychiatry-your-brain-on-food-201511168626.

Shukla, Apoorva, Sonali G. Choudhari, Abhay M. Gaidhane, and Zahiruddin Quiza Syed. 2022. "Role of Art Therapy in the Promotion of Mental Health: A Critical Review." *Cureus* 14(8): e28026. Accessed on December 25, 2024. https://doi.org/10.7759/cureus.28026.

Smith, Sara. "5-4-3-2-1 Coping Technique for Anxiety," *University of Rochester Medical Center*, April 10, 2018. Accessed on December 20, 2024. https://www.urmc.rochester.edu/behavioral-health-partners/bhp-blog/april-2018/5-4-3-2-1-coping-technique-for-anxiety.

Snijders, Clara, Lotta-Katrin Pries, Noemi Sgammeglia, Ghazi Al Jowf, Nagy A. Youssef, Laurence de Nijs, Sinan Goluksuz, and Bart P.F. Rutten. 2018. "Resilience Against Traumatic Stress: Current Developments and Future Directions." *Frontiers in Psychology* 9: 676. Accessed on December 27, 2024. https://doi.org/10.3389/fpsyt.2018.00676.

Spritzler, Franziska. "9 Side Effects of Too Much Caffeine," *Healthline*, June 21, 2023. Accessed on December 27, 2024. https://www.healthline.com/nutrition/caffeine-side-effects.

Stathokostas, Liza, Robert M. D. Little, A. A. Vandervoort, and Donald H. Paterson. 2012. "Flexibility Training and Functional Ability in Older Adults: A Systematic Review." *Journal of Aging Research* 2012: 306818. Accessed on December 21, 2024. https://doi.org/10.1155/2012/306818.

Stevens, Suzanne. "Imagery Rehearsal Therapy Can Help You Rewrite Nightmares for Sweeter Sleep," *Healthline*, August 19, 2022. Accessed on December 21, 2024. https://www.healthline.com/health/sleep/imagery-rehearsal-therapy.

Stinson, Adrienne. "What is Box Breathing?," *Medical News Today*, May 13, 2024. Accessed on December 20, 2024. https://www.medicalnewstoday.com/articles/321805.

Terlizzi, Emily P. and Jeannine S. Schiller. 2022. "Mental Health Treatment Among Adults Aged 18–44: United States, 2019–2021." NCHS Data Brief No. 444. National Center for Health Statistics. Accessed on December 18, 2024. https://doi.org/10.15620/cdc:120293.

Vernor, Dale. "PTSD is More Likely in Women Than Men," *National Alliance on Mental Illness*, October 8, 2019. Accessed on December 24, 2024. https://www.nami.org/stigma/ptsd-is-more-likely-in-women-than-men/.

von Bernhardi, Rommy, Laura Eugenín-von Bernhardi, and Jaime Eugenín. 2017. "What Is Neural Plasticity?" *Advances in Experimental Medicine and Biology* 1015: 1-15. Accessed on December 18, 2024. https://doi.org/10.1007/978-3-319-62817-2_1.

Wadyka, Sally. "The Link Between Highly Processed Foods and Brain Health," *New*

*York Times*, August 1, 2024. Accessed on December 21, 2024. https://www.nytimes.com/2023/05/04/well/eat/ultraprocessed-food-mental-health.html.

West, Kathleen E., Michael R. Jablonski, Benjamin Warfield, Kate S. Cecil, Mary James, Melissa A. Ayers, James Maida, Charles Bowen, David H. Sliney, Mark D. Rollag, John P. Hanifin, and George C. Brainard. 2011. "Blue Light From Light-Emitting Diodes Elicits a Dose-Dependent Suppression of Melatonin in Humans." *Journal of Applied Physiology* 110(3): 619-26. Accessed on December 21, 2024. https://doi.org/10.1152/japplphysiol.01413.2009.

West, Mary. 2022. "What to Know About Guided Imagery," *Medical News Today*, April 21. Accessed on December 27, 2024. https://www.medicalnewstoday.com/articles/guided-imagery.

"Violence Against Women," World Health Organization, March 25, 2024. Accessed on December 18, 2024. https://www.who.int/news-room/fact-sheets/detail/violence-against-women.

Yu, Jie, Zhenqing Yang, Sudan Sun, Kaili Sun, Weiran Chen, Liming Zhang, Jiahui Xu, Qinglin Xu, Zuyun Liu, Juan Ke, Lisan Zhang, and Yubo Zhu. 2024. "The Effect of Weighted Blankets on Sleep and Related Disorders: A Brief Review." *Frontiers in Psychiatry* 15: 1333015. Accessed on December 21, 2024. https://doi.org/10.3389/fpsyt.2024.1333015.

Made in the USA
Las Vegas, NV
20 March 2025